# MAKING SENSE OF THE CHEST X-RAY

# MAKING SENSE OF THE CHEST X-RAY

## A HANDS-ON GUIDE

**Paul F. Jenkins**
MA MB BChir FRCP(London) FRCP(Edinburgh)
Consultant Physician, Norfolk and Norwich University Hospital
NHS Trust, Norwich, UK

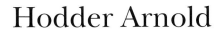

Hodder Arnold

A MEMBER OF THE HODDER HEADLINE GROUP

First published in Great Britain in 2005 by
Hodder Education, a member of the Hodder Headline Group,
338 Euston Road, London NW1 3BH

http://www.hoddereducation.com

Distributed in the United States of America by
Oxford University Press Inc.,
198 Madison Avenue, New York, NY 10016
Oxford is a registered trademark of Oxford University Press

Whilst the advice and information in this book are believed to be true and
accurate at the date of going to press, neither the author[s] nor the publisher
can accept any legal responsibility or liability for any errors or omissions
that may be made. In particular, (but without limiting the generality of the
preceding disclaimer) every effort has been made to check drug dosages;
however it is still possible that errors have been missed. Furthermore,
dosage schedules are constantly being revised and new side-effects
recognized. For these reasons the reader is strongly urged to consult the
drug companies' printed instructions before administering any of the drugs
recommended in this book.

British Library Cataloguing in Publication Data
A catalogue record for this book is available from the British Library

Library of Congress Cataloging-in-Publication Data
A catalog record for this book is available from the Library of Congress

ISBN-10 [normal]:     0 340 88542 4
ISBN-13 [normal]:     978 0 340 88542 0
ISBN-10 [ISE]:        0 340 88557 2
ISBN-13 [ISE]:        978 0 340 88557 4
                      (International Students' Edition, restricted territorial availability)

1 2 3 4 5 6 7 8 9 10

Commissioning Editor: Joanna Koster
Project Editor: Heather Smith
Production Controller: Jane Lawrence
Cover Design: Sarah Rees
Illustrations: Cactus Design and Illustrations Ltd

Index: Indexing Specialists (UK) Ltd

Typeset in 10.5/13 Rotis Serif by Charon Tec Pvt. Ltd, Chennai, India
Printed and bound in Italy

What do you think about this book? Or any other Hodder Arnold title?
Please visit our website at www.hoddereducation.com

# CONTENTS

# PREFACE

This book is not intended to provide an exhaustive reference
for differential diagnosis based on the chest radiograph.
Instead, I offer a practical approach to chest X-ray
interpretation, which may be of use to doctors and other
healthcare professionals who need to develop these techniques
as part of their assessment, diagnosis and management of
patients. The chest radiograph is an immensely valuable tool
in clinical medicine and to be proficient in its interpretation is
a fundamental skill for clinicians. It is also a skill that is
intensely intellectually satisfying and I hope that these pages
and the illustrations I have selected will encourage your
enthusiasm for its development. A further reading list is
appended, comprising texts that are on my shelves and
including some that have been there for more years than
I will admit to!

I have emphasized a problem-solving approach throughout
the book, an approach whereby an observation stimulates
active questioning and a search for ancillary radiographic
appearances, in an attempt to narrow the differential
diagnosis by collating maximum information from the
image.

For example, there may be an area of consolidation in right
mid-zone and the sequence of questioning, which follows, is:

● how well circumscribed is the shadowing?
● how dense is it (soft tissue or denser)?

- is there an air-bronchogram within it?
- can I see cavitation ?
- does the shadow 'cross fissures'?
- is there associated pleural disease, bone disease or lymphadenopathy?

Being aware of the questions to ask and seeking to answer them in a proactive, inquisitorial manner expedites diagnosis. As far as the above example is concerned, systematic questioning may suggest that consolidation is secondary to proximal bronchial obstruction rather than being due to simple infection, therefore raising the possibility of bronchial carcinoma and emphasizing the need to consider early bronchoscopy in this patient's management.

In this way, the practical approach I describe should contribute to speedy and efficient clinical management. Look at Figs 1 and 2.

Figure 1 shows an alveolar-filling pattern in the mid-zones, in peri-hilar distribution. There is of course a differential

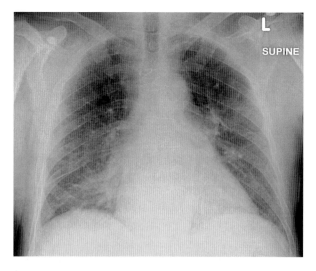

Figure 1

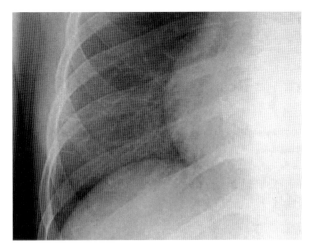

Figure 2

diagnosis here and this includes pulmonary oedema, pulmonary alveolar haemorrhage, adult respiratory distress syndrome, pneumonia and so on. In fact, any pathological process, which can result in alveolar filling should be considered in the initial differential diagnosis. However, the sequence of questioning outlined above results in the ancillary observations of a small right pleural effusion, fluid in the lesser fissure, cardiomegaly and septal lines at the bases (shown beautifully in close-up in Fig. 2). With this combination of features, one can be confident of the diagnosis of left heart failure. The presence of sternal sutures is additional evidence of heart disease.

A chest radiograph in isolation is limited in its contribution to diagnosis, and its usefulness is enhanced tremendously when it is interpreted in conjunction with knowledge of the clinical findings. A collaborative diagnostic approach is therefore encouraged throughout the book and I have used a 'clinical association' icon to emphasize this partnership. Remember also though that a chest radiograph, just like any other test, has to be requested for a reason, and if performed must be looked at. These statements seem self-evident but surveys have questioned doctors' discrimination before asking for a radiographic investigation and have also described significant numbers of X-rays that have not been promptly interpreted after they have been performed.

I have also used icons to emphasize potential pitfalls in interpretation, interesting points to ponder and 'pearls of wisdom'!
The icons used are as follows:

● Clinical association

● Hazard

● Thinking point

● 'Pearl of wisdom'

Finally, I have sought out illustrations that commonly show more than one abnormality. This is intentional and is designed to bring continual emphasis to one of the basic themes of the book, namely the need to interpret the radiograph systematically and thereby acquire all of the information it has to offer in diagnosis and management. **The examination is not complete when one abnormality has been discovered.**

# ACKNOWLEDGEMENTS

Much of the detailed discussion in this book has evolved
from the problem-solving teaching sessions I have led over
the years and I am immensely indebted to those whom I have
taught because I have learnt so much from them.

I am also deeply in debt to two ex-bosses of mine, Drs Dewi
Davies and Roderick Smith who were consultants in
Nottingham when I was a registrar there. Their enthusiasm
and wisdom stimulated my desire to be a chest physician.
Dewi taught me the discipline of rigid clinical observation
(he was responsible for much original descriptive writing)
and Roderick allowed me to glimpse the combination of
huge clinical astuteness with genuine humility. They were
delightful personalities who provided role models I have
never forgotten – offering standards to be aspired to if not
achieved.

John Curtin is a chest radiologist here in Norwich and has
been enormously helpful in seeking out illustrations for
this book. I am very grateful to him for this and for his wise
counsel over the investigation of many patients in the past.

This book is dedicated to my two sons, David and Peter and
to my wife Glynis. Glyn has had to endure its conception
and development and that cannot have been easy. It is also
dedicated to my parents, my father who saw me qualify and
my mother who, sadly, didn't. Without their guidance and

support I would never have had the opportunity of joining such a fantastic profession.

If readers derive half as much pleasure from reading *Making Sense of the Chest X-ray* as I have in writing it (and especially if fewer radiographic mistakes are made at the 'front-door' as a result), then I will consider the book a success.

# LIST OF ABBREVIATIONS

| | |
|---|---|
| ARDS | adult respiratory distress syndrome |
| ASD | atrial septal defect |
| BHL | bilateral hilar lymphadenopathy |
| COPD | chronic obstructive pulmonary disease |
| CT | computerized tomography |
| CTPA | computerized tomography (CT) pulmonary angiogram |
| CWP | coal-workers' pneumoconiosis |
| CXR | chest X-ray |
| ECG | electrocardiogram |
| ESR | erythrocyte sedimentation rate |
| JVP | jugular venous pressure |
| $P_aCO_2$ | arterial carbon dioxide tension |
| $P_ACO_2$ | alveolar carbon dioxide tension |
| $P_aO_2$ | arterial oxygen tension |
| $P_AO_2$ | alveolar oxygen tension |
| PCP | *Pneumocystis carinii* pneumonia |
| $P_IO_2$ | oxygen tension in inspired air |
| PMF | progressive massive fibrosis |
| PTB | pulmonary tuberculosis |
| $S_aO_2$ | arterial oxygen saturation |
| SARS | severe acute respiratory syndrome |
| SBE | standard base excess |
| TR | tricuspid regurgitation |

# 1

# THE SYSTEMATIC APPROACH

Be disciplined and train yourself to follow a system when interpreting a chest radiograph. Examine anatomical structures in strict order because if you deviate from this systematic approach, you risk missing important information, particularly if your eye is drawn by the obvious abnormality and further critical examination is overlooked. I recall someone falling into this trap recently when he considered the diagnosis complete after describing multiple rounded shadows on a chest radiograph. These were well-defined, of variable sizes and obviously represented metastatic malignant disease. Unfortunately, he did not notice the right mastectomy, which was clearly present and the likely source of the metastatic deposits. He had not adopted a systematic approach to interpretation of the image in front of him and had failed to look at the breast shadows specifically. In the past, I have missed osteolytic lesions in ribs for exactly the same reason.

Always follow a system and continually ask yourself specific questions on the observations you make. Of course, 'pattern recognition' is a vital part of chest radiograph interpretation and it will become increasingly so as you become more experienced, but never allow yourself to abbreviate the systematic approach.

Here is the system I follow:

## BASIC OBSERVATIONS FIRST

● Note the patient's name, age and ethnic background. These details may provide clues as to the possible diagnosis.

● What is the date of the radiograph? It contributes far more to patient care if you make a stunning diagnosis on an X-ray that is current rather than on one that is two years old.

● Has the radiograph been taken in postero-anterior or antero-posterior projection? If the latter, then it is impossible to comment accurately on heart size.

● How centred is the image? Look at the sterno-clavicular joints when making this assessment and you will see from Fig. 1.1 (a normal chest radiograph) that the right and left joints are equidistant from the mid-line. This is a well-centred radiograph. A rotated film will

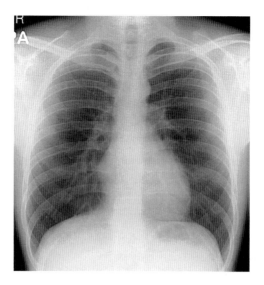

**Figure 1.1** Normal chest X-ray.

adversely affect the interpretation of all anatomical structures, particularly those within the mediastinum – in fact, evaluation may be impossible if the image is significantly skewed.

● Next decide on the degree of radiographic penetration of the image. Basically, ideal penetration applies when you can see vertebral bodies clearly through the heart shadow. Sometimes a softer film helps in defining pulmonary infiltration and, in these days of digital images, it is possible to manipulate the window level in order to optimize penetration. Figure 1.1 is an example of near-perfect X-ray penetration.

● Finally, examine the alignment of the ribs. Figure 1.2 shows the horizontal appearance of the ribs, apparent when a radiograph has been taken in a lordotic (leaning back) position.

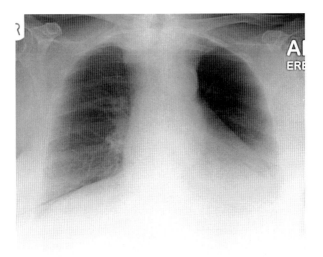

**Figure 1.2** The horizontal appearance of the ribs, apparent when a radiograph has been taken in a lordotic (leaning back) position.

Figure 1.3 illustrates the characteristic acute angle between posterior and lateral ribs in the patient with pectus

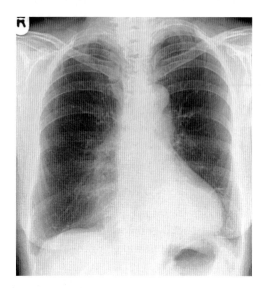

**Figure 1.3** The characteristic acute angle between posterior and lateral ribs in a patient with pectus excavatum.

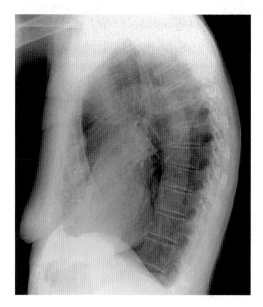

**Figure 1.4** The same patient as in Fig.1.4 X-rayed in the right lateral position.

excavatum. Note the 'fuzziness' adjacent to the right heart border, which is a normal accompaniment of this anatomical variant. Recognition of 'pectus' from the shape of the rib cage will negate the concern that there might be consolidation in right middle lobe. Figure1.4 shows the same patient X-rayed in right lateral position, and the pectus is clearly seen.

You are now ready to start examining specific areas, continually asking questions of the appearances you detect:

## START IN THE NECK

- Is the trachea deviated or compressed? If so, this is compatible with retrosternal thyroid enlargement (Fig. 1.5).
- Can you see surgical emphysema in the soft tissues of the neck? Figure 1.6 is an obvious example in a young person

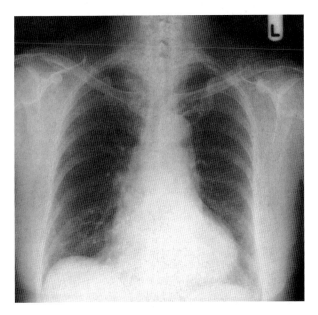

**Figure 1.5** Retrosternal thyroid goitre showing indentation and deviation of the trachea.

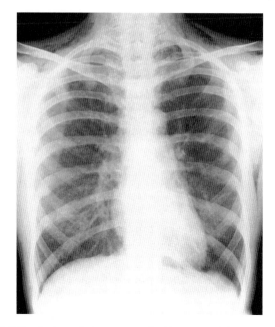

**Figure 1.6** Surgical emphysema complicating acute asthma.

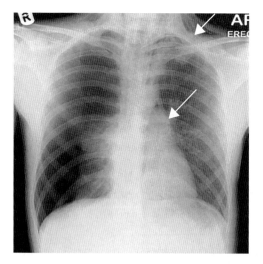

**Figure 1.7** Pneumothorax and pneumomediastinum. Note the air in the soft tissues of the neck as well as the line defining the left mediastinal structures (both arrowed).

with an acute attack of asthma but the appearances are often very subtle and will be missed unless you look for them specifically.

Interestingly, one cannot see a pneumomediastinum in Fig.1.6 although presumably there is one. Figure 1.7, on the other hand shows obvious air in the mediastinum in association with a tension pneumothorax. With this combination it is vital to consider the possibility of oesophageal rupture – in this case though, air had leaked from an apical bulla in this young man's right lung. Surgical emphysema can be seen clearly in the neck.

## HAZARD

It is important to diagnose pneumomediastinum. Asthmatics rarely come to harm from this complication of acute asthma but air in the mediastinum can also result from oesophageal rupture and this condition must not be missed. Spontaneous rupture of the oesophagus does happen. It is usually associated with an episode of vomiting but the severity of the vomiting can be surprisingly slight.

## CLINICAL CONSIDERATIONS

The classical physical signs of pneumomediastinum are palpable surgical emphysema in the neck and Hamman's sound. This is a crunching noise heard over the praecordium, throughout the cardiac cycle, similar to, though more 'crackly' than, a pericardial rub.

● Is there tell-tale calcification in the area of the thyroid gland, typical of a thyroid adenoma?
● Are cervical ribs evident? These can be responsible for neurological symptoms due to nerve entrapment (Fig. 1.8).

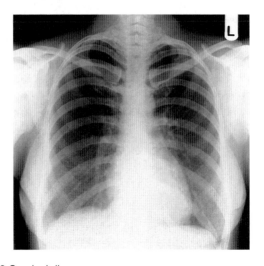

**Figure 1.8** Cervical ribs.

## Examine the mediastinal structures

● Is the aortic root of normal size? If it is small, this may indicate an atrial septal defect (ASD; Fig. 1.9). The

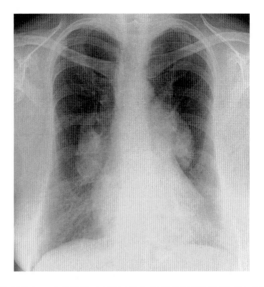

**Figure 1.9** Atrial septal defect; all of the radiographic features are shown as described in the text.

ancillary radiographic appearances of this diagnosis are prominent hilar shadows and exaggerated vascular markings in the lung fields, appearances that will be recorded if your systematic 'problem solving' is up to scratch.

 **CLINICAL CONSIDERATIONS**

Clinical confirmation of an ASD relies on the classical physical signs of a pulmonary flow murmur, a fixed and split second heart sound and a flow murmur in mid-diastole across the tricuspid valve.

If the aortic root is prominent, the commonest reasons are hypertension or degenerative unfolding of the aorta. Sometimes, though, prominence is indicative of thoracic aortic dissection – the 'double-shadow' in the aortic arch, described as suggestive of aortic dissection is an uncommon finding (Figs 1.10 and 1.11).

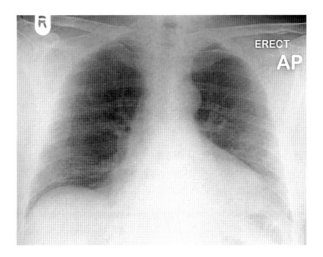

**Figure 1.10** Aortic dissection with a normal chest X-ray.

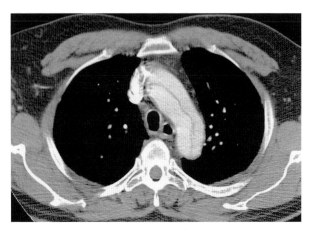

**Figure 1.11** The CT scan of the patient in Fig. 1.10.

 **HAZARD**

A normal appearance of the aortic arch on chest X-ray (CXR) does not exclude an aortic dissection. If this diagnosis is suspected, computerized tomography (CT) and/or trans-oesophageal echocardiography is mandatory.

 **CLINICAL CONSIDERATIONS**

The diagnosis should be suspected if chest pain is described as tearing in nature, of sudden onset and, especially, if it is felt predominantly in the back.

Proceed down the left mediastinal border, investigating as follows:

● Is the left hilum of normal size and shape and in the correct position? The left hilum should be slightly higher

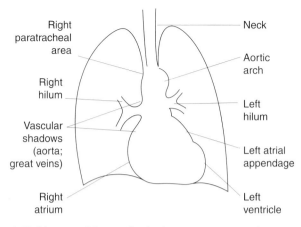

**Figure 1.12** Diagram of the mediastinal structures to examine on posterior–anterior chest X-ray.

than the right on posterior–anterior (p–a) view (Fig. 1.12) and any change in position of either is suggestive of loss of volume in the respective lung field.

For example, upward 'shift' of the left hilum is a cardinal feature of loss of volume in left upper lobe and the bilateral upper zone fibrosis of post-primary tuberculosis is associated with upward shift of both hila (Fig. 1.13). (The concept of 'shift of normal structures' in identifying areas of pulmonary collapse is expanded in Chapter 4.)

Deciding whether a hilum is normal or enlarged and, if the latter, whether this is due to exaggerated pulmonary vessels or hilar lymphadenopathy is not easy, but knowledge of a few basic facts and a systematic approach helps tremendously. This is discussed further in Chapter 2.

● Just below the left hilar shadow is the area, which, if prominent, suggests enlargement of the left atrial appendage as part of left atrial enlargement. This is less common nowadays but was hitherto typically associated with rheumatic mitral valve disease (Fig. 1.14).

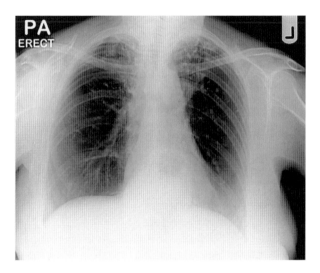

**Figure 1.13** Bilateral upward hilar shift as a result of tuberculosis.

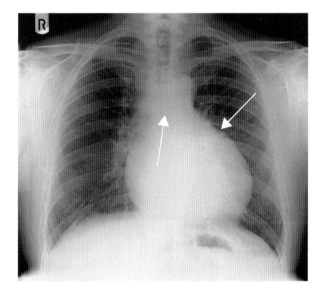

**Figure 1.14** Left atrial enlargement. Note the prominence of the left atrial appendage, and 'splaying' of the main carina, which are both arrowed.

## CLINICAL CONSIDERATIONS

Listen carefully for the murmurs of mitral valve disease.

- Continue by examining the left ventricular contour. Cardiomegaly is indicative of ventricular dilatation associated with volume overload (aortic or mitral valve regurgitation), primary left ventricular disease (ischaemic or due to a cardiomyopathy) or pericardial effusion (Figs 1.15 and 1.16).

Calcification can occasionally be seen in the outline of the left ventricle and this is indicative of previous myocardial infarction with or without aneurysm formation (Fig. 1.17)

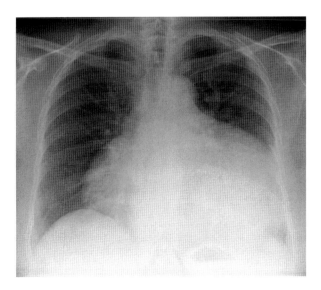

**Figure 1.15**  Chest radiograph showing pericardial effusion. Note the characteristic shape of both right and left heart borders.

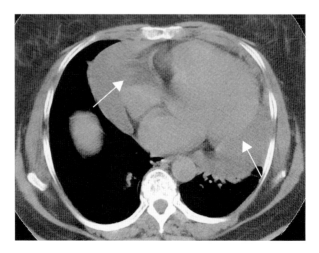

**Figure 1.16** CT appearances in the same patient; the pericardial fluid is arrowed.

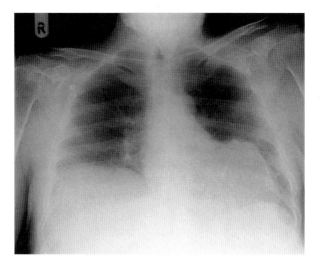

**Figure 1.17** A thin rim of calcium in an old myocardial infarct which has become aneurysmal.

● Now turn your attention to the right mediastinal structures, starting with the right heart border. This normally represents the right atrial shadow and if it is enlarged to the right may indicate tricuspid regurgitation (TR).

**CLINICAL CONSIDERATIONS**

The clinical signs of TR are:

- 'V' waves (or, more strictly, 'S'– systolic – waves) in the neck
- an expansile liver
- a pansystolic murmur, heard best at the left sternal edge but often fairly unimpressive.

- The right heart border continues with the ascending aorta, abnormal prominence of which occurs as a result of degenerative unfolding as well as with aneurysm formation.
- Is the right hilum normally positioned and of normal size?
- Examine the paratracheal area. Lymphadenopathy here is characteristically associated with right hilar enlargement, plus or minus left hilar enlargement in the mediastinal lymphadenopathy of sarcoidosis (Fig. 1.18).

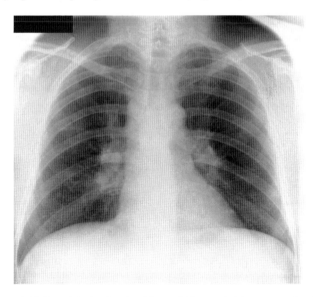

**Figure 1.18** Sarcoidosis showing bilateral hilar and right paratracheal lymphadenopathy.

You have now successfully completed the 'mediastinal circuit'! There is much more regarding specific mediastinal pathology in Chapter 2.

## NOW TURN YOUR ATTENTION TO THE PLEURAL REFLECTIONS

Start by examining each hemidiaphragm in turn and working your way laterally and upwards to each lung apex. Look carefully and ask specific questions; it is so easy to miss calcified asbestos pleural plaques on the hemidiaphragms unless you question their presence specifically (Fig. 1.19).

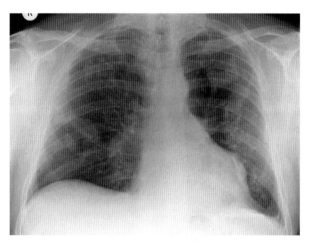

**Figure 1.19** Calcified asbestos pleural plaque on left hemidiaphragm.

Figure 1.19 also shows the characteristic pleural calcification of asbestos plaques overlying the right and left lung fields. This is the so-called 'holly-leaf' pattern and, although this romantic description is sometimes quite optimistic, Fig. 1.20 is a superb example and vindicates the analogy.

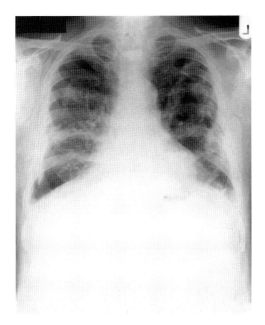

**Figure 1.20** 'Holly-leaf' pattern of calcified asbestos plaques.

## PEARL OF WISDOM

Asbestos fibres travel to the periphery of the lung, perforate visceral pleura and set up an inflammatory reaction as visceral and parietal pleura rub together during the respiratory cycle. The irritative effect is facilitated by contiguous solid structures and this explains why asbestos plaques develop characteristically on the hemidiaphragms as well as laterally as they follow the contours of the ribs.

## THE PENULTIMATE STEP IN YOUR CIRCUIT IS TO CONCENTRATE ON THE LUNG FIELDS

Examine and compare the lung apices, the upper zones, mid-zones and lower zones in turn.

Look specifically for:

● differences in density
● the possibility of pulmonary infiltration
● evidence of an alveolar-filling process.

Always do your best to explain visible lines. A line in the right mid-zone may indicate a thickened or fluid-filled fissure and if there is loss of volume in right lower lobe, the right oblique fissure may become visible to the X-ray beam as the shrinking lobe moves posteriorly and medially. Figure 1.21 shows these changes in diagrammatic form.

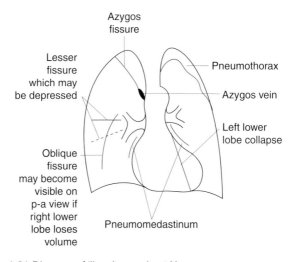

**Figure 1.21** Diagram of 'lines' on a chest X-ray.

A peripheral line may indicate a pneumothorax (Fig. 1.22) and a line parallel to part of the mediastinum may be the only clue to the presence of a pneumomediastinum (Fig. 1.7, page 6). Figures 1.23 and 1.24 are examples of other lines, which require explanation.

These are all clear examples of their respective pathologies but be aware that the appearances are very often less dramatic and you should be alert to subtle changes (Fig. 1.25).

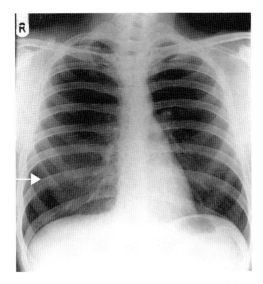

**Figure 1.22** Right-sided pneumothorax in a young man. The edge of the lung is arrowed.

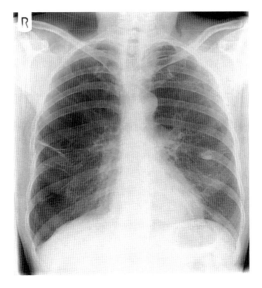

**Figure 1.23** Emphysematous bullae in a 44-year-old smoker. There is a granuloma in the left mid-zone and note the vascular changes of pulmonary hypertension.

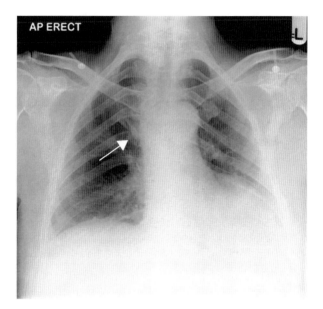

**Figure 1.24** The characteristic appearance of an azygos lobe, with the lozenge-shaped azygos vein at its inferior extremity (arrowed).

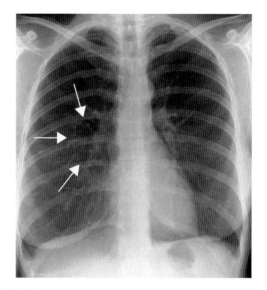

**Figure 1.25** Subtle line shadow outlining an emphysematous bulla (arrowed).

## YOU HAVE NOT QUITE FINISHED

It is good discipline to return to examine four areas specifically, four areas that are easy to overlook:

### Behind the heart

Be sure not to miss a hiatus hernia. The enormous incarcerated hiatus hernia shown in Fig. 1.26 is obvious but that in Fig. 1.13 is far less so. Similarly learn to look for the tell-tale line of left lower lobe collapse (Fig. 1.27) and look specifically for a mass behind the heart. Figure 1.28 shows a neural tumour in this area and you will see how easy it is to overlook the abnormality on a p–a chest radiograph. In contrast, the subsequent CT scan (Fig. 1.29) was striking.

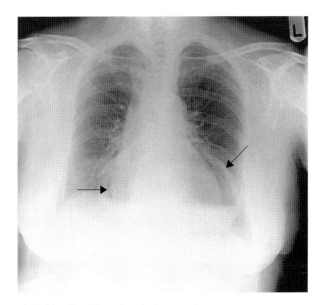

**Figure 1.26** Massive hiatus hernia (arrowed).

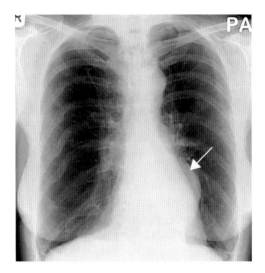

**Figure 1.27** Left lower lobe collapse with the responsible bronchial carcinoma arrowed as a visible mass. Note old fractures of right ribs. These were unrelated and had followed a nasty fall some years previously.

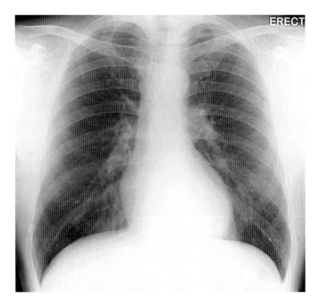

**Figure 1.28** Neurogenic tumour posterior to the heart.

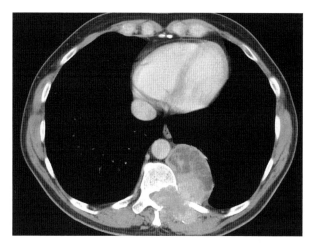

**Figure 1.29** CT scan of Fig. 1.28. Neurogenic tumour posterior to heart. This was a malignant peripheral nerve sheath tumour.

 **PEARL OF WISDOM**

When looking behind the heart, try turning the image back-to-front. Your colleagues may think that you are demented but, strangely, it is often easier to see posterior shadows in this way.

## Breast shadows

If you do not look specifically, sooner or later you will fail to remark on a mastectomy. Figure 1.30 is more subtle; the breasts are of very different shapes and this lady has undergone right lumpectomy with subsequent radiotherapy. Note also the loss of volume in right upper lobe with upward shift of right hilum and lesser fissure (arrowed). Unhappily, an endobronchial secondary deposit had developed in right upper lobe bronchus. This was suspected radiographically after she presented acutely with cough and dyspnoea, and the diagnosis was subsequently confirmed at bronchoscopy.

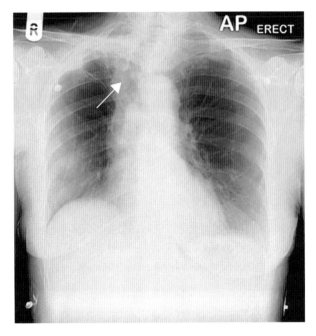

**Figure 1.30** Previous 'lumpectomy' of the right breast. Also collapse of right upper lobe, due to an endobronchial secondary deposit.

Radiotherapy resulted in excellent symptom improvement and the patient is alive three years after this CXR was performed.

## Below the diaphragm

Look specifically for air below the diaphragm (Figs 1.31 and 1.32). This young man had a perforated duodenal ulcer.

Very rarely, one can see calcification within the liver due to hydatid cyst or within the spleen, indicative of splenic infarction secondary to sickle-cell disease. I did have wonderful examples of both but as someone has 'borrowed' the films I am afraid and I will have to settle for an abdominal radiograph showing a calcified hydatid cyst in the mesentery (Fig. 1.33).

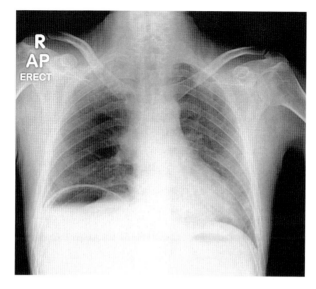

**Figure 1.31** This young man had a perforated duodenal ulcer. Note the right hilar lymphadenophy – he also had non-Hodgkin's lymphoma.

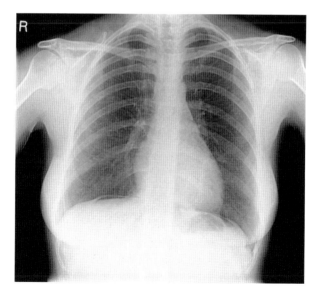

**Figure 1.32** The changes are more subtle in this young lady who had undergone recent abdominal surgery.

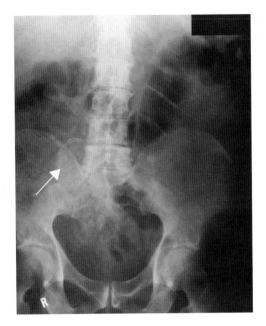

**Figure 1.33** A calcified mesenteric hydatid cyst (arrowed).

## Bones

Look at **all** bony structures very carefully – this includes the clavicles, upper arms, shoulder joints etc.

Figure 1.34 shows rib destruction in association with a pancoast tumour.

 **CLINICAL CONSIDERATIONS**

This patient had a Horner's syndrome on the right.

Figure 1.35 shows generalized sclerosis in the ribs, clavicles and upper arms due to metastatic prostatic carcinoma.

Figure 1.36 shows an enormously expanding lytic lesion in a left rib.

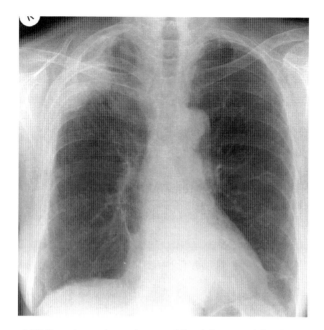

**Figure 1.34** Bronchogenic carcinoma of the right upper lobe destroying the right 3rd rib.

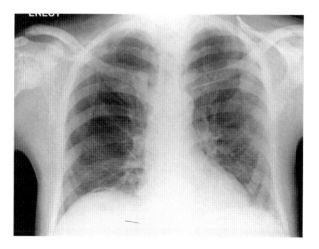

**Figure 1.35** Sclerotic bone metastases from prostate cancer. Free air under the right hemidiaphragm is due to a perforated gastric ulcer.

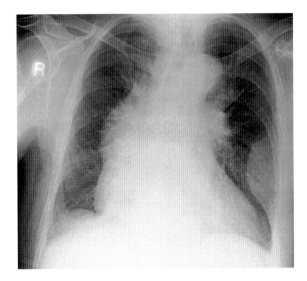

**Figure 1.36** This 83-year-old man has a lytic rib lesion with an unknown primary – note the expanding deposit. The left hilum looks suspicious. The ascending aorta was unfolded and not aneurysmal.

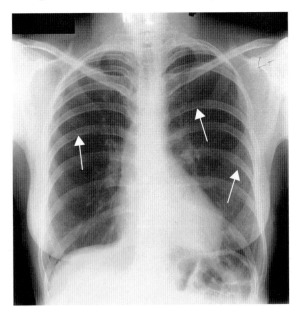

**Figure 1.37** Corrected coarctation of the aorta in a young woman. The characteristic 'rib-notching' is arrowed.

Figure 1.37 is a striking example of rib-notching in a young woman who had had correction of coarctation of the aorta. Note the missing left fifth rib, the legacy of her lateral thoracotomy.

Finally:

 **PEARL OF WISDOM**

It is easier to look at the ribs if you turn the image on its side with the relevant ribs uppermost. Honestly, it works.

Your systematic examination of the chest radiograph is now complete and it is time to move on to specific areas of interest.

# 2

# MEDIASTINAL AND HILAR SHADOWS

Mediastinal and hilar abnormalities offer a significant challenge. They may be difficult to see on a chest radiograph and it is vital to follow a system such as that outlined in Chapter 1. The differential diagnosis of mediastinal abnormalities is complex but, despite this, a knowledge of the possible causes of abnormal shadowing in each of the mediastinal 'geographical departments', superior, anterior, middle and posterior, helps tremendously in differentiating pathology and this is discussed later. I think it is useful to start with a few tips in answering the common and potentially difficult question, 'is this hilum abnormal?'.

## THE 'BULKY' HILUM

Let's consider some basic points first of all:

● In a healthy person the hilar shadows are created by the pulmonary arteries and veins with a small contribution from the walls of the major bronchi. The latter appear as narrow line shadows outlined on the one hand by the air contained within them and on the other by adjacent aerated lung. They can often be seen on a well-exposed radiograph and an intrabronchial obstructing lesion (carcinoma or foreign body, for example) can encroach on these line shadows – an appearance that is particularly helpful if there is associated lobar collapse.

It is a useful exercise to take some simple measurements of the basal arteries when assessing the size of the hila (Fig. 2.1). Each basal artery tapers distally and, on the right, a convenient, though arbitrary, point to measure the artery is at its mid-point. The measurement is taken from its lateral wall to the transradiancy of the intermediate bronchus medially. This is shown in the diagram as distance '*y*' and varies in normal middle-aged adults between 7 and 19 mm with a mean of 14 mm.

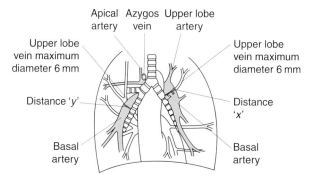

Pulmonary arteries shaded, pulmonary veins unshaded

**Figure 2.1** Hilar shadows and measurements. Distance '*x*' = 18–32 mm (average 24 mm); distance '*y*' = 7–19 mm (average 14 mm). Pulmonary arteries are shaded, pulmonary veins are unshaded.

 **CLINICAL CONSIDERATIONS**

If this transradiant area at the medial wall of the right basal artery is lost on a well-centred radiograph it may suggest non-vascular pathology within, or adjacent to, the right hilum.

When assessing the left hilum, measurement '*x*' is taken from the point where the left upper lobe bronchus crosses behind the basal artery and from the latter's medial wall to its superior border. In normal adults this distance measures 18–32 mm (mean 24 mm; Fig. 2.1).

Quantifying the size of the hilar shadows in this way does result in a more objective assessment than the totally subjective, 'I think this hilum looks prominent' approach.

It is also useful to have clear landmarks for identifying the normal position of each hilum. In Fig. 2.1, the lines '$x$' and '$y$' start superiorly where the most lateral upper lobe vein meets the basal arteries. If this point is taken as the centre of each hilum, on the right it will be opposite the horizontal fissure (which meets the 6th rib in the axilla), or roughly at the level of the 3rd rib anteriorly on deep inspiration. On the left, the centre of the hilum is 0.5–1.5 cm higher. Using these landmarks it becomes possible to determine movement of the hilar shadows in an objective way.

 **PEARL OF WISDOM**

A final word about measurement. The normal upper lobe pulmonary veins where they meet the upper border of their respective basal artery (Fig. 2.1) have diameters of 4–6 mm. They are enlarged in pulmonary venous congestion due to heart failure or mitral valve disease.

- An abnormally prominent hilum is either caused by exaggerated vascular shadowing or by pathological enlargement of non-vascular structures and you should attempt to distinguish between the two possibilities:
  - first, remember the clinical point above regarding preservation of the transradiant area medial to the right basal artery and representing air within the intermediate bronchus
  - second, focus on a shadow that is obviously vascular at the edge of the hilum and follow it back into the hilar shadow. Continue to dissect the hilar structures in this way and then decide if you are left with any component of this shadow which cannot be explained on the basis of exaggerated vascular structures.

Neither of these tips is infallible but they are a quick and easy evaluation unless the image is rotated, in which case interpretation may be impossible.

Figure 2.2 is the radiograph of a lady with Eisenmenger's syndrome. Using the principles just discussed we can be confident of the vascular nature of the huge hilar shadows. ('$x$' measures 50 mm and '$y$' measures 45 mm)

Figure 2.3 also shows prominent hila due to vascular enlargement. This lady has pulmonary hypertension as a result of chronic obstructive pulmonary disease.

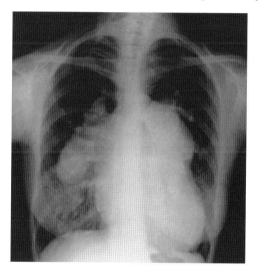

**Figure 2.2**
Eisenmenger's syndrome with enormous enlargement of the pulmonary vessels.

Figure 2.4 is an example of bilateral hilar lymphadenopathy (BHL) in sarcoidosis. Although the medial border of the right basal artery is still outlined, the 'lumpiness' of both hilar

  **HAZARD**

Note also the abnormal shape of the right breast and the clips in the right axilla in Fig. 2.3. This patient had had a carcinoma of the breast treated surgically and with

radiotherapy. There are healing fractures of ribs 3, 4, 5 and 6 and fortunately these were caused by trauma and were not metastatic. Only a systematic approach will ensure that all of these abnormalities are detected.

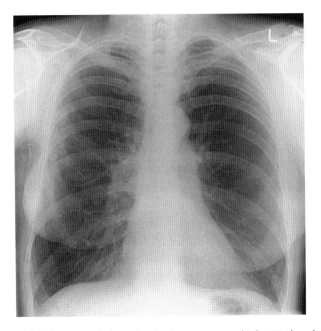

**Figure 2.3** Enlargement of proximal pulmonary vessels due to chronic obstructive pulmonary disease in a lady who has had treatment for carcinoma of the right breast.

shadows is not comfortably explained by simple vascular prominence. Figure 2.5 emphasizes this point as a more florid example of sarcoid-related BHL.

● Additionally, look for ancillary clues of pathology on the radiograph. Figure 2.6 illustrates paratracheal lymphadenopathy and multiple patches of consolidation in the lung fields as well as right hilar enlargement. This man had long-standing sarcoidosis. Other examples of ancillary abnormalities are a peripheral mass

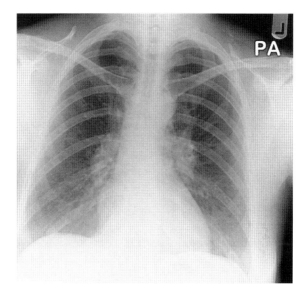

**Figure 2.4** Sarcoidosis, showing bilateral hilar lymphadenopathy.

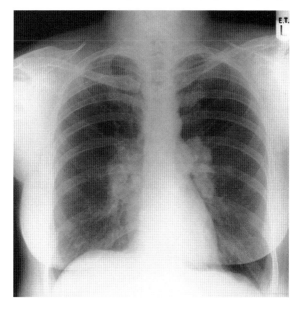

**Figure 2.5** A more florid example of bilateral hilar lymphadenopathy due to sarcoidosis.

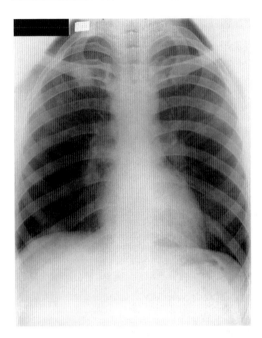

**Figure 2.6**
Bilateral hilar lymphadenopathy, paratracheal lymph node enlargement and multiple areas of pulmonary infiltration in a case of sarcoidosis.

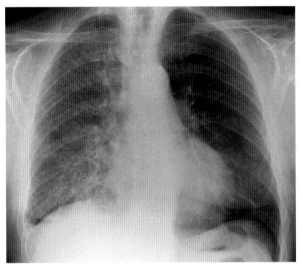

**Figure 2.7** Lymphangitis carcinomatosa and a small right pleural effusion. The hilar glands were very enlarged and preceded the intrapulmonary appearances. The primary carcinoma was in the breast.

(a real give-away as far as diagnosis is concerned), a pleural effusion or perhaps lymphangitis in association with hilar lymph node enlargement (Fig. 2.7).

● Most often, one is questioning whether a hilum may be abnormally large but, occasionally, one or other hilum may be smaller than normal. This is seen (together with generalized hyperlucency of the lung on the same side) in Macleod's syndrome and occasionally in other situations (Fig. 2.8).

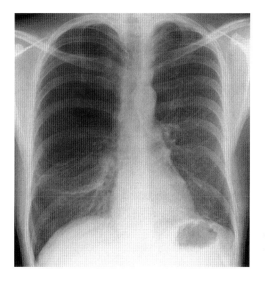

**Figure 2.8** An apparently small right hilum, which is also pushed downward by a large emphysematous bulla.

 **PEARL OF WISDOM**

**Macleod's syndrome:** Swyer and James in 1953 and then Macleod, in 1954, described unilateral hyperlucent lung and this condition is ascribed to severe neonatal or childhood bronchiolitis resulting in destruction of lung units at a time when their numbers are developing. Chest radiography is diagnostic with the combination of a normal-sized or small lung, which is hyperlucent, and ipsilateral pulmonary vessels that are small and distributed sparsely throughout the lung field.

# CAUSES OF HILAR ENLARGEMENT

## Vascular

We have seen examples of prominent proximal vascular markings as a feature of established pulmonary hypertension (the commonest cause of which is chronic obstructive pulmonary disease) and in congenital heart disease. Unilateral hilar vascular enlargement can occur in massive pulmonary embolism when it may be seen in association with hyperlucency of part of the ipsilateral lung field (Westermark's sign).

## Non-vascular

**THINKING POINT**

Let's now consider non-vascular pathology, and when we do it is important to understand that in these conditions hilar lymphadenopathy is regularly accompanied by enlargement of other groups of intrathoracic lymph nodes and that the pattern of distribution of this enlargement can help in pathological diagnosis.

*Lymph node enlargement caused by lymphoma and leukaemia*

Mediastinal lymph node enlargement is the most common radiographic finding in Hodgkin's disease and is seen on the initial chest radiograph of approximately 50 per cent of patients with this condition. In the majority, lymph node involvement is bilateral though asymmetric. Unilateral node enlargement is unusual. Paratracheal and subcarinal nodes are involved as often as, or even more often than, hilar nodes. Interestingly, involvement of anterior mediastinal and retrosternal nodes is common, and this anatomic distribution is a major factor in distinguishing lymphoma from sarcoidosis – sarcoidosis rarely causes radiographically visible nodal enlargement in the anterior mediastinal compartment.

Mediastinal and/or hilar lymph node enlargement is also the commonest intrathoracic manifestation of non-Hodgkin's lymphoma and of leukaemia. Not surprisingly, leukaemic lymphadenopathy is far commoner in the lymphocytic forms of this disease.

### Metastatic lymph node enlargement

Lymphomas are responsible for the majority of mediastinal lymph node malignancies but the second most common cause of lymph node enlargement is metastasis from solid tumours, especially from the lungs, upper gastrointestinal tract, prostate, kidneys and genitals.

---

> **?** **THINKING POINT**
>
> When the primary lesion is in the lung, nodal enlargement is almost always unilateral. Also, the primary lesion may be barely visible or even invisible, a situation highly suggestive of an 'oat-cell' primary (Fig. 4.51, page 131).

---

### Lymph node involvement in granulomatous diseases

This category includes infective causes such as tuberculosis and histoplasmosis (rare in this country but more common in the US) as well as sarcoidosis.

In the infectious granulomas, lymphadenopathy tends to be predominantly unilateral (Fig. 2.9). This isn't universal and Fig. 2.10 shows symmetrical bilateral hilar lymphadenopathy in a child with primary tuberculosis.

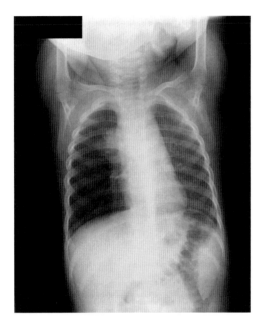

**Figure 2.9**
Unilateral right hilar
and paratracheal
lymphadenopathy in
a Chinese child with
primary tuberculosis.

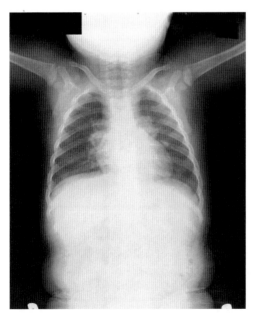

**Figure 2.10**
A Caucasian child
with primary
tuberculosis. The
hilar nodes are
symmetrically
enlarged.

Hilar lymphadenopathy in sarcoidosis is usually bilateral (Fig. 2.5), although the right hilar nodes are commonly more prominent.

### PEARL OF WISDOM

Very importantly, mediastinal lymph node enlargement in sarcoidosis is almost invariably associated with hilar node involvement and this is an important differentiating feature from lymphoma.

### THINKING POINT

If lymph nodes are calcified this is highly suggestive of an infective or granulomatous cause although the characteristic 'egg-shell' calcification of sarcoidosis is also seen in silicosis (Figs 2.11 and 2.12).

*Unusual causes of mediastinal lymphadenopathy*

● Lymph node hyperplasia was originally described by Castleman in 1954. The X-ray appearance is of a solitary mass with a smooth or lobulated contour in any of the three mediastinal compartments and most commonly in the middle and posterior ones. Although these masses can grow very large, they seldom cause symptoms and the histological appearance is typical and non-malignant. It has been suggested that the condition represents a hamartoma of lymphoid tissue.
● Infectious mononucleosis is a rare cause of mediastinal and hilar lymphadenopathy.

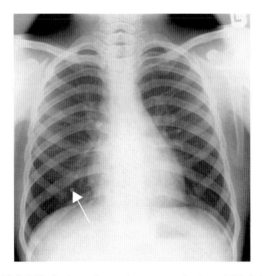

**Figure 2.11** Calcified tuberculous primary complex in a child. At least one Ghon focus can be seen (arrowed) as well as the calcified right hilar nodes.

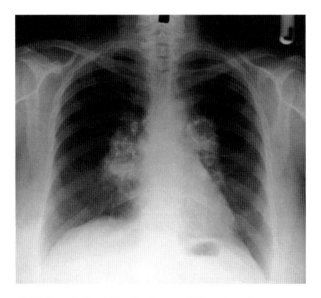

**Figure 2.12** Egg-shell calcification in sarcoid lymph nodes.

# MEDIASTINAL GEOGRAPHY

The anatomical boundaries of the mediastinum are the thoracic inlet superiorly, the diaphragm inferiorly and the parietal pleura (investing the medial surfaces of the lungs) on both sides laterally.

Figure 2.13 is a diagrammatic representation, shown in left lateral view, of three hypothetical mediastinal areas and the organs contained within them.

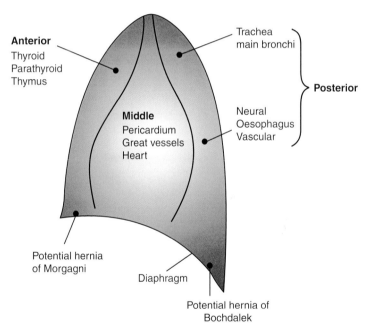

**Figure 2.13** Diagrammatic representation of the mediastinum seen in left lateral view, showing the organs residing in the anterior, middle and posterior compartments respectively.

● The anterior compartment is bounded by the sternum anteriorly, the pericardium posteriorly and the diaphragm inferiorly.

**Table 2.1** Mediastinal masses, tabulated according to compartment (see text)

| Anterior compartment | Middle compartment | Posterior compartment | More than one compartment |
|---|---|---|---|
| Retrosternal thyroid | Pericardial cyst | Neural tumour | Lymphoma |
| Thymic masses | Aortic aneurysm | Oesophagus | Metastatic solid tumour |
| • hyperplasia | Anomalous or ectatic vessels | • tumour | Sarcoidosis |
| • cyst | Left ventricular aneurysm | • achalasia | Tuberculosis |
| • thymoma | Cardiomegaly | • gastroenteric cyst | Castleman's disease |
| Germ cell tumours | | Trachea | Bronchial and gastroenteric |
| • benign (dermoid) | | • bronchogenic cyst | cysts |
| • malignant | | Hiatus hernia | |
| Lymphoma | | Bochdalek hernia | |
| Other malignancies | | Descending aorta | |
| Morgagni hernia | | aneurysm | |

- The anterior boundary of the posterior compartment is the posterior surface of the pericardium. Posteriorly it abuts on the vertebral bodies and the paravertebral gutters and, inferiorly, it reaches the diaphragm.
- The middle compartment is bounded by the pericardium.
- The three compartments come together and become less well defined in the superior mediastinum.

The division of the mediastinum into anterior, middle and posterior compartments in this way, together with consideration of the tumour masses, which may be expected in each one (Table 2.1), is a valuable exercise in arriving at a differential diagnosis of abnormal mediastinal shadowing.

## Some examples of mediastinal masses

Figure 2.14 shows a large retrosternal thyroid goitre with concentric narrowing of the trachea. The extent of the narrowing is shown dramatically in Fig. 2.15, which is a computerized tomography (CT) scan of the same patient.

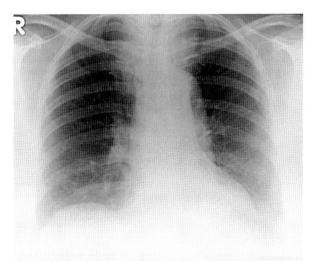

**Figure 2.14** Retrosternal thyroid goitre surrounding and narrowing the trachea.

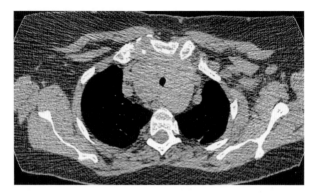

**Figure 2.15** CT scan of the patient in Fig. 2.14, showing dramatic concentric narrowing of the trachea.

Figures 2.16 and 2.17 are the chest radiograph and CT scan, respectively, of a young man with Hodgkin's lymphoma. Comparing this chest radiograph with Fig. 2.14, you can see a more defined upper border whereas the thyroid mass continues up to and merges with thoracic inlet.

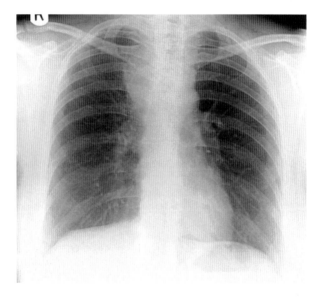

**Figure 2.16** Lymphoma creating a right paratracheal mass.

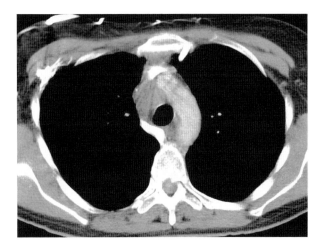

**Figure 2.17** CT scan of the patient shown in Fig. 2.16.

The bronchogenic cyst illustrated in Figs 2.18 and 2.19 has a different shape again. In all fairness, one could not reliably differentiate this from lymphoma on the chest radiograph alone, and the CT scan is more reassuring of its benign nature.

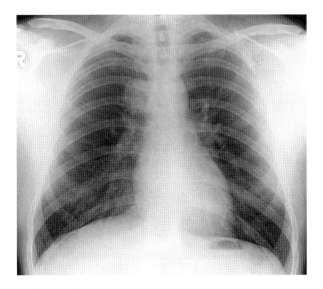

**Figure 2.18** Bronchogenic cyst.

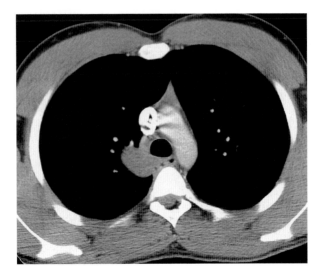

**Figure 2.19** CT scan of bronchogenic cyst in Fig. 2.18.

The anterior mediastinal mass clearly seen in Fig. 2.20 developed in a middle-aged lady who had myasthenia gravis. It is no surprise then that this proved to be a thymoma. Figure 2.21 is a CT scan from the same patient.

The young man whose chest X-ray is shown in Fig. 2.22 presented with chest pain. The posterior–anterior radiograph is fairly unimpressive but the CT scan (Fig. 2.23) is highly abnormal, showing a large anterior mediastinal mass, which turned out to be caused by a teratoma.

 **PEARL OF WISDOM**

**Teratoma:** Sometimes, unusual tissue elements including bone can be seen in these germinal cell tumours.

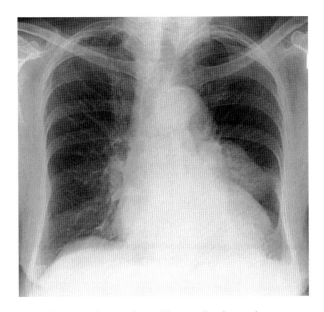

**Figure 2.20** Thymoma in a patient with myasthenia gravis.

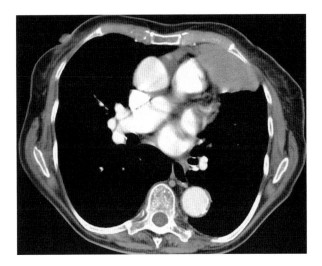

**Figure 2.21** CT of patient depicted in Fig. 2.20.

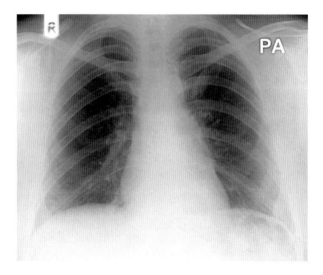

**Figure 2.22** Teratoma in a young man. The anterior mediastinal mass is difficult to see on chest radiograph but the area adjacent to the left hilum looks very suspicious.

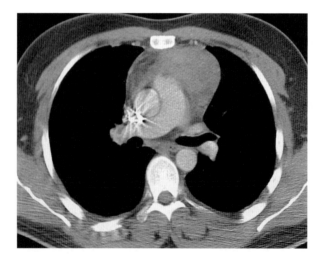

**Figure 2.23** CT scan of the young man in Fig. 2.22.

There are no prizes for diagnosing the cause of the anterior mediastinal mass shown on chest radiograph in Fig. 2.24 and subsequent CT scan in Fig. 2.25, but . . .

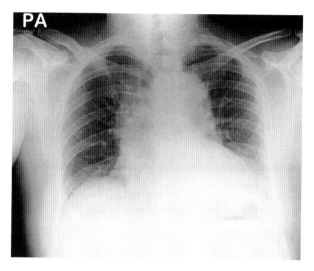

**Figure 2.24** Aortic dissection with a widened mediastinum.

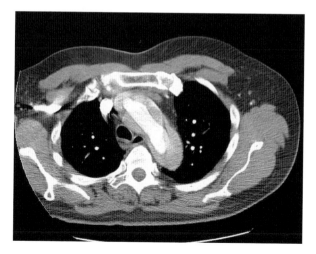

**Figure 2.25** CT scan of the patient in Fig. 2.24.

## CLINICAL CONSIDERATION

. . . these images belonged to a 55-year-old man who presented with severe chest pain that radiated to his back. There was an aortic diastolic murmur on auscultation and the clinical findings together with the chest radiograph secured the diagnosis of aortic dissection. Happily, he has made an excellent recovery following surgery and prompt diagnosis was crucial in ensuring this.

Identifying posterior mediastinal masses can be difficult, particularly if the shadowing is behind the heart and I take you back to Figs 1.28 and 1.29 (pages 22 and 23) in order to illustrate the point.

We are going to leave the mediastinum now and the next two chapters concentrate on aspects of abnormal intrapulmonary shadowing.

# 3

# CONSOLIDATION, COLLAPSE AND CAVITATION

This chapter discusses the radiographic patterns of pulmonary consolidation and illustrates the various pathological processes that can cause it. It also describes the features of partial and complete loss of volume of the major lobes of the lungs.
We are all aware that it may be difficult to decide if there is abnormal parenchymal shadowing on a chest radiograph and most of us will have missed subtle changes of lobar collapse at some stage in our careers as well. There is a systematic approach to the identification of both consolidation and collapse, however, and in this Chapter, I seek to share it.
I guarantee that if the system is adopted and practised then eventually 'pattern recognition' will take over – in other words, 'I have seen this lots of times before and I know what it is'. Before any of us reaches this stage of experience, however, it is vital to be obsessional about our systematic approach – but then this applies to all aspects of clinical medicine.

## DEFINITIONS

### Consolidation

Consolidation is a pathological term. It describes the state of the lung when alveolar gas has been replaced by fluid, cells or a mixture of the two. Various terms have been used in an attempt to describe the morphological appearance of consolidation and these include 'alveolar-filling pattern', 'airspace filling' and 'ground-glass shadowing'. I prefer the first of these because it is so descriptive and I use it preferentially in this chapter.

Whatever the terminology, the radiographic appearances of consolidation are those of homogeneous shadowing in part of the lung field with little or no lobar shrinkage. The normal vascular pattern is lost because the alveolar-filling process denies the definition of lung markings by replacing the air in adjacent lung parenchyma. This loss of vascular pattern is a major clue when the appearances of consolidation are subtle.

What none of these terms can determine though is the pathological nature of the substance that has resulted in alveolar filling. They do not differentiate between pneumonic infiltrate and the transudate of heart failure, and they cannot distinguish alveolar haemorrhage from *Pneumocystis carinii* pneumonia or the malignant infiltrate of alveolar cell carcinoma. However, there are additional clues on a radiograph that can narrow the pathological diagnosis and one should always seek these out. As an example, the distribution of consolidation in eosinophilic pneumonia, which is described as, 'reverse pulmonary oedema' can be virtually diagnostic with predominantly peripheral consolidation not confined to individual lobes or segments (Figs 3.1 and 3.2).

Another example, as discussed in Chapter 1, is the association of an alveolar-filling pattern with pleural effusions, cardiomegaly and interstitial lines, which virtually secures the diagnosis of heart failure.

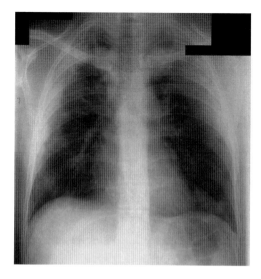

**Figure 3.1** Peripheral consolidation in eosinophilic pneumonia.

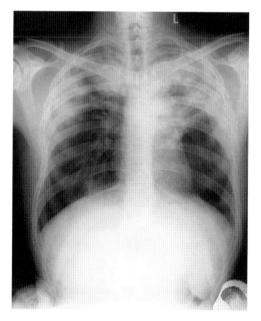

**Figure 3.2** Another example of eosinophilic pneumonia.

**CLINICAL CONSIDERATIONS**

Heart failure is usually associated with cardiomegaly but not exclusively so. Normal heart size may be retained under the following circumstances:

- if heart failure is of sudden onset. The classic example is mitral valve rupture after myocardial infarction
- sometimes in restrictive cardiomyopathies
- more rarely with pericardial disease
- with mitral valve disease. In the days of rheumatic fever, mitral stenosis regularly progressed to cause left **atrial** failure, the X-ray manifestations of which are the same as left ventricular failure.

These days, of course, the additional information available from high-resolution computed tomography (CT) scanning is particularly enlightening in determining the cause of consolidation.

## Collapse

Consolidated lung may lose volume at any stage in its natural history but the crucial question is whether consolidation is secondary to collapse (the classical cause being major airway obstruction), because this has important management implications – marked loss of volume on the radiograph is likely to indicate pathology causing primary collapse and should be investigated as such.

When the primary process is consolidation, on the other hand, any subsequent loss of volume isn't usually dramatic unless the disease is a chronic infective one like tuberculosis or chronic *Klebsiella* pneumonia. One of the reasons for emphasizing this point is to question the value of the compromise term 'consolidation-collapse'. To use this description seems scarcely worthwhile because it does not assist in deciding the presence or absence of bronchial occlusion and, therefore, does not materially guide patient management.

## Density

When referring to radiographic shadowing, the term 'density' refers to the radio-opacity of a lesion and this will be influenced fundamentally by the degree of exposure of the film. With this important qualification and assuming ideal radiographic exposure of the image, I think it is useful to consider three grades of density as follows:

● **low density**: small shadows caused by cells or body fluids
● **medium density**: larger shadows especially caused by fluids
● **high density**: shadows containing radio-opaque atoms either derived from body fluids (iron or calcium) or introduced from the environment (iron, calcium, barium or tin).

Inevitably, these distinctions will be subjective to a certain extent and, in particular, the separation of low- and medium-density shadows can be difficult, but the classification is still helpful and I would recommend it to you.

## A SYSTEMATIC APPROACH TO CONSOLIDATION (OR ALVEOLAR FILLING)

### Ensure that the abnormal shadowing represents an alveolar-filling process

Pulmonary infiltrates of various sorts can become heavy and coalesce so that they mimic 'alveolar filling' – examine the nature of the shadowing carefully. Is it truly homogeneous or does it appear to be a coalescence of rounded shadows (nodular), streaky shadows (reticular) or a combination of the two (reticulo-nodular)? The intrapulmonary shadowing in Fig. 3.3 is certainly generalized and may appear homogeneous at first sight. However, closer inspection reveals that it is made up of myriads of tiny dots in all areas of the lung fields – it almost looks as though someone has scattered the contents

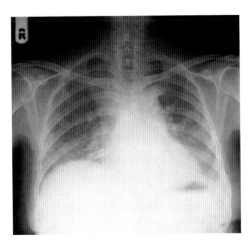

**Figure 3.3** Miliary tuberculosis.

of a salt-cellar over the film. This elderly lady had fatal miliary tuberculosis.

## What is the distribution of the abnormal shadowing?

Lobar pneumonia affects lobes or segments uniformly (Figs 3.4 and 3.5). Pneumonia caused by a variety of infecting agents, including the pneumococcus, can affect multiple lobes or segments but the radiographic appearance of multiple segmental or subsegmental consolidation should arouse diagnostic suspicion of non-infective aetiology:

● if the shadowing is predominantly peripheral, eosinophilic pneumonia should be considered (Fig. 3.6). Early suspicion is easy if the X-ray shows classical 'reverse pulmonary oedema' but this isn't always the case
● the corollary to this is that other non-infective but inflammatory conditions cause multisegmental consolidation. Figure 3.7 is an example of cryptogenic organizing pneumonitis, an inflammatory condition whose clinical presentation also commonly mimics pneumonia. It is a condition that also requires treatment with corticosteroids.

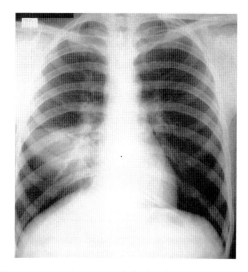

**Figure 3.4** Pneumococcal pneumonia in the right middle lobe. The consolidation has a sharp upper boundary where it abuts the lesser fissure. The heart border is lost, confirming this as anterior shadowing and therefore confined to the middle lobe. Air-bronchogram was absent.

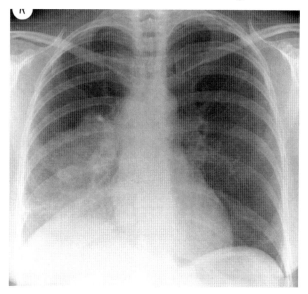

**Figure 3.5** Pneumococcal pneumonia in the right lower lobe. This time the heart border is preserved, the upper boundary is indistinct but the right hemidiaphragm is blurred.

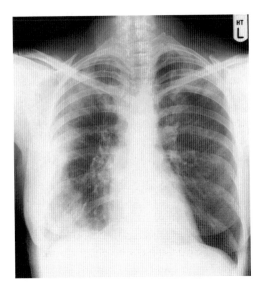

**Figure 3.6** Eosinophilic pneumonia with predominance of right-sided shadowing, though this is still very peripheral.

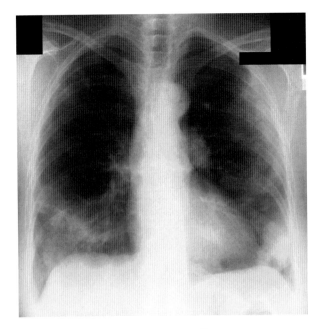

**Figure 3.7** Cryptogenic organizing pneumonitis.

## CLINICAL CONSIDERATIONS

Figure 3.7 is interesting because a lot of the shadowing is peripheral and our initial diagnosis was that of eosinophilic pneumonia. The correct diagnosis was made on lung biopsy.

- Wegener's granulomatosis is a vasculitic disease, which characteristically produces multiple areas of consolidation when it affects the lungs. These lesions commonly cavitate (Fig. 3.8).
- Rarely, sarcoidosis can produce multisegmental areas of consolidation. I have heard the term, 'clouds of Turieff' used to describe the rather macronodular pattern illustrated in Fig. 3.9 but I have not seen this eponymous title in any of the more modern texts. Figure 3.10 shows areas of consolidation but there are nodules as well.

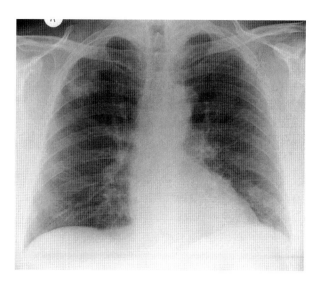

**Figure 3.8** Wegener's granulomatosis: right upper lobe and left lower lobe lesions. There is a hint of cavitation in the former.

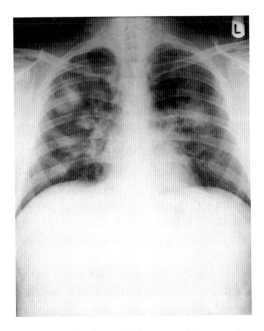

**Figure 3.9** Sarcoidosis showing multiple segmental areas of consolidation.

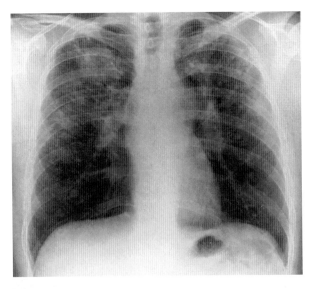

**Figure 3.10** Sarcoid: with nodules and areas of consolidation.
The bilateral hilar lymphadenopathy is a clue to the diagnosis.

- Malignant infiltrates (haematological, lymphoproliferative and solid tissue tumours) are also in the differential diagnosis of 'multisegmental consolidation'.

 **HAZARD**

The fundamental message is to consider non-infective pathology if there are multiple areas of consolidation. A thorough interpretation of the radiograph will raise your suspicions and help to ensure early appropriate treatment because, even though the story may sound like infection, this radiographic pattern can be caused by disease processes that will not respond to antibiotics.

Other recognizable radiographic patterns include:

- pulmonary oedema has a characteristic peri-hilar distribution and the epithet, 'bat's-wing of death', though unfortunate, is often appropriate morphologically (Fig. 3.11)

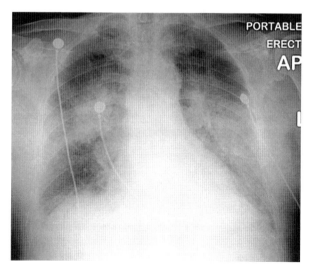

**Figure 3.11** Pulmonary oedema; the 'bat's-wing' appearance.

- bilateral consolidation in the lower zones may suggest aspiration pneumonia, and loss of volume may be associated because bronchial obstruction due to aspirated material is a real possibility
- alveolar haemorrhage is commonly peri-hilar in distribution but this isn't totally reliable, e.g. the major haemorrhage shown in Fig. 3.12 has resulted in extensive bilateral consolidation. Note that there is no air-bronchogram within the shadowing because blood is filling the airways as well as the alveoli.

In contrast:

- there are no distinguishing radiographic features displayed by the bilateral alveolar-filling pattern in this example of pulmonary alveolar proteinosis (Fig. 3.13) and the same applies to most cases of *Pneumocystis carinii* pneumonia (Fig. 3.14) and alveolar cell carcinoma (Fig. 3.15).

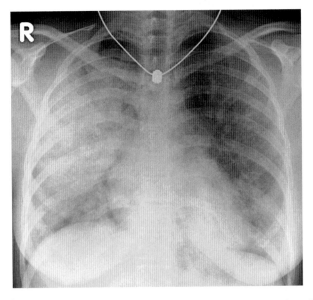

**Figure 3.12** Extensive alveolar haemorrhage in a patient with idiopathic pulmonary haemosiderosis.

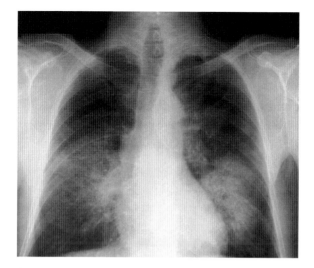

**Figure 3.13** Pulmonary alveolar proteinosis.

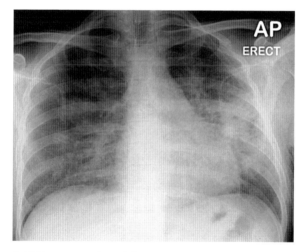

**Figure 3.14** *Pneumocystis carinii* pneumonia in a patient with acquired immune deficiency syndrome (AIDS). Extensive bilateral alveolar-filling pattern.

The consolidation in Fig. 3.16 is in a patient with the adult respiratory distress syndrome and, although the multitude of tubes and wires may be a clue as to aetiology, there is nothing diagnostic about the radiograph *per se*.

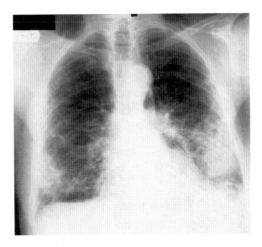

**Figure 3.15** The consolidation in this case was due to alveolar cell carcinoma.

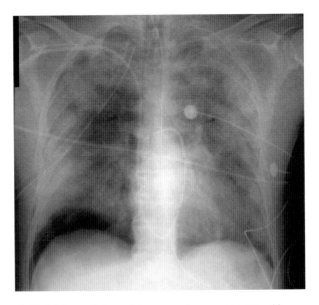

**Figure 3.16** Adult respiratory distress syndrome complete with pulmonary flotation catheter, nasogastric and endotracheal tubes, intercostal chest drain and electrocardiogram wires.

## THINKING POINT

The basic learning point accruing from the last four cases is that although lungs become consolidated in a variety of pathological conditions the radiographic appearance of 'alveolar filling' is ubiquitous and non-discriminatory in many instances.

## What is the density of the shadowing?

Sometimes, consolidation is of low density, but more commonly it is medium dense, representing as it does alveoli filled with fluid, cells, infective organisms or a mixture of these components. Heavy density shadowing is not seen except under unusual circumstances, e.g. if a radio-dense foreign body is responsible for bronchial obstruction.

## CLINICAL CONSIDERATIONS

I remember just this situation in a middle-aged man with a heavy alcohol intake who presented one weekend extremely septic with pneumonia. He had consolidation with no air-bronchogram in right middle and lower lobes and there appeared to be a calcified area approximately 1 cm$^2$ in right mid-zone. I bronchoscoped him that night and retrieved a vertebral body of a small mammal (presumably a rabbit) from the intermediate bronchus. He recovered remarkably well despite the fact that *Actinomyces* was present in bronchial aspirate. He had no recollection of consuming said mammal!

- When cavitation is seen in an area of consolidation it indicates either a particular infecting organism (*Staphylococcus*, mycobacteria and Gram-negative organisms should be in your differential; Figs 3.17 and 3.18), bronchial

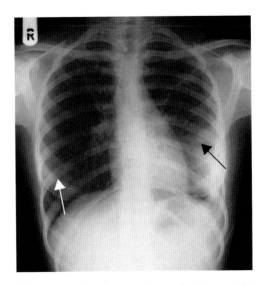

**Figure 3.17** There are bilateral areas of consolidation on this young girl's radiograph. Several of them are starting to cavitate (arrowed). *Staphylococcus* was the infecting organism.

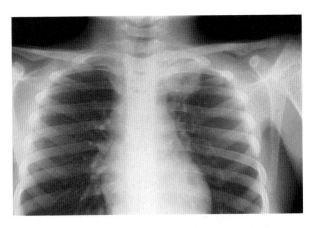

**Figure 3.18** The single area of apical consolidation in this child has an obvious cavity. This was progression of primary tuberculosis.

obstruction with distal cavitation (complicating a bronchial carcinoma (Fig. 3.19) or foreign body), or a completely different pathological process, e.g., primary lung abscess (Fig 3.20) or a cavitating pulmonary infarct.

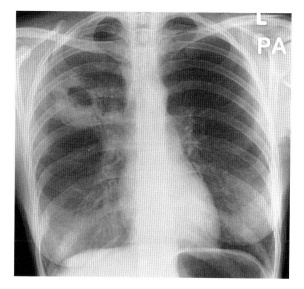

**Figure 3.19** This 65-year-old lady had a cavitating squamous cell carcinoma.

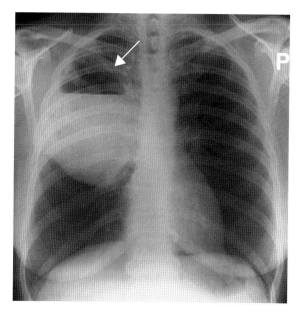

**Figure 3.20** This was a primary lung abscess. Note the thick upper walls (arrowed).

## Is there an associated 'air-bronchogram'?

An air-bronchogram is created by the persistence of air-filled bronchi travelling through an area of consolidated lung, looking like the branches of a tree after autumn's leaf-fall. Figure 3.21 is an example though not quite as dramatic as the romantic seasonal analogy!

---

### ? THINKING POINT

The presence or absence of an air-bronchogram provides clues as to the underlying pathology. When absent, it indicates that the airways have become filled with material of equivalent radio-density to that of the surrounding consolidated lung. Absence of an air-bronchogram in association with extensive consolidation suggests either an infective process with large amounts of secretions – the classic examples being pneumococcal or staphylococcal pneumonia (Fig. 3.4, page 59) – or consolidation in association with proximal bronchial obstruction – carcinoma, foreign body, aspiration and so on (Figs 3.22 and 3.23).

---

## Is there radiographic evidence of other disease?

The obvious associated abnormalities to look for are lymphadenopathy, bony pathology (Fig. 3.24) or pleural shadowing.

---

###  CLINICAL CONSIDERATIONS

A unilateral pleural effusion in the presence of consolidation can suggest an underlying malignancy or perhaps indicate empyema formation. Both of these possibilities demand investigation, commencing with diagnostic pleural aspiration with or without pleural biopsy.

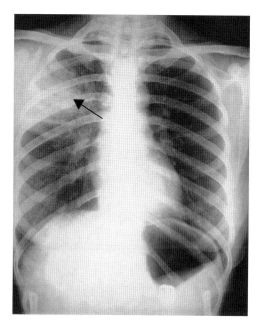

**Figure 3.21** An air-bronchogram (arrowed) can be clearly seen in this radiograph of pneumococcal pneumonia affecting the posterior segment of the right upper lobe.

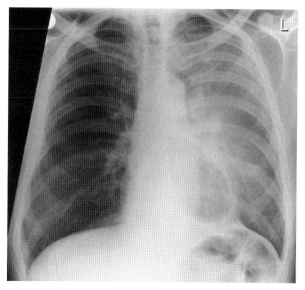

**Figure 3.22** Left upper lobe consolidation (and a minor degree of collapse). There is no air-bronchogram. Note the large hiatus hernia. This was aspiration pneumonia with obstruction to the left upper lobe bronchus.

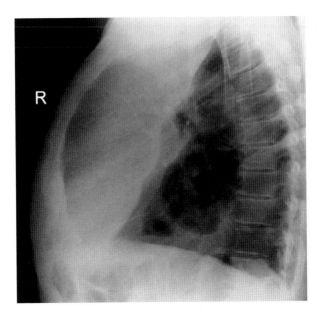

**Figure 3.23** Lateral view of Fig. 3.22.

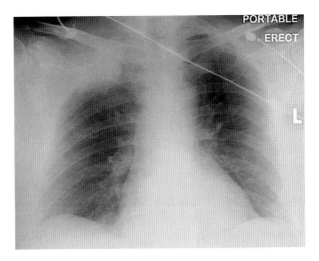

**Figure 3.24** Pancoast tumour destroying 1st and 2nd ribs.

**CLINICAL CONSIDERATIONS**

Unilateral pleural effusion does occur in pulmonary oedema but bilateral effusions are more typical though quite commonly asymmetric in size.

## Is there significant associated loss of volume?

If so this is highly suggestive of underlying, often malignant, disease and this observation may well dictate the need for early bronchoscopic investigation.

Let's move on to consider a diagnostic approach to pulmonary collapse.

## COLLAPSE

An important part of this discussion is to look at examples of collapse of all the major lobes and I suggest their repeated examination in order to engender 'pattern recognition'. In addition, there are some basic points to consider:

● If a lobe has collapsed completely, it may be radiographically invisible. Figure 3.25 is an example; an occluding bronchial carcinoma has resulted in total collapse of right upper lobe, which has virtually disappeared. Under these circumstances, one has to rely on ancillary radiographic changes to make the diagnosis and I will discuss these in a little while.

● On the other hand, complete collapse of the left lower lobe almost invariably leaves a characteristic line behind the heart and this appearance should stimulate you to search for confirmatory radiographic signs of loss of volume in this lobe (Fig. 3.26).

● A lateral chest radiograph can be very useful in confirming major collapse, particularly of the middle lobe and lingula (Figs 3.34 and 3.37, pages 80 and 82, respectively) but in

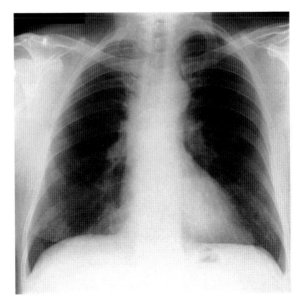

**Figure 3.25** Complete collapse of right upper lobe.

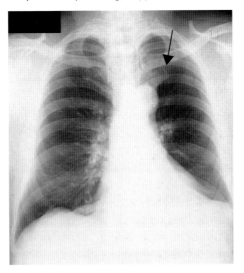

**Figure 3.26** Left lower lobe collapse. Note the calcified tuberculous lymph nodes in the mediastinum (behind the aortic knuckle) and the hila. The latter clearly illustrate the downward shift of the left hilum. Finally note the Ghon focus at the left apex (arrowed).

other instances it can be disappointingly unhelpful and this applies especially to the lower lobes (Fig. 3.27).

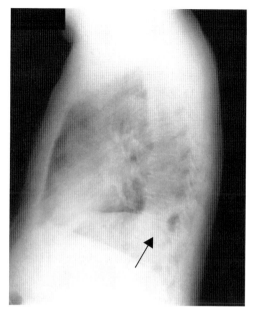

**Figure 3.27** Left lateral view of Fig. 3.26. This is fairly unremarkable but the clues to left lower lobe pathology are the left elevated hemidiaphragm and the shadow superimposed on vertebral bodies (arrowed).

## The radiographic signs of collapse

There are three categories of radiographic signs that contribute to the recognition of lobar collapse:

1  The shadow created by the abnormal lobe itself. As we have seen, this may be of little help if the offending lobe has collapsed completely.
2  Loss of normal lines and shadows. The lines created by anatomical structures will become blurred if abnormal, non-aerated lung collapses against them. For example, the medial part of the respective hemidiaphragm becomes indistinct in the presence of collapse of one or other lower lobe (Figs 3.38 and 3.39, page 83). Similarly, there is loss

(or blurring) of the respective heart border in middle lobe or lingula collapse (Figs 3.33, 3.35 and 3.36, pages 80, 81 and 82), the paravertebral structures become indistinct in lower lobe collapse (Figs 3.38 and 3.39, page 83) and so does the right upper mediastinum in right upper lobe collapse. This is illustrated well in Fig. 3.25.

3   'Shift of normal structures'. The hilar shadows are pulled downwards by corresponding lower lobe collapse and upwards by shrinking upper lobes.

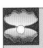 **PEARL OF WISDOM**

The middle lobe is interesting When it loses volume, the lesser fissure and the right oblique fissure move together though the former tends to move more (Fig. 3.34, page 80). The hilum can move downward slightly therefore, but when it can be seen to have moved significantly this indicates combined right middle and right lower lobe collapse, a picture that strongly suggests obstruction in the intermediate bronchus. Similarly, one or other hemidiaphragm may move upward in association with lobar collapse (Figs 3.32 and 3.39, pages 79 and 83, respectively) and mediastinal structures can shift to the same side if there is major hemithoracic loss of volume, particularly with complete lung collapse (Fig. 3.28). This feature is crucial in distinguishing collapsed lung from massive pleural effusion in unilateral 'white-out' (Chapter 5: Pleural disease).

## Examples of lobar collapse
*Right upper lobe*

Complete collapse (Fig. 3.25) results in blurring of the right upper mediastinal shadows and upward shift of the right hilum. The lobe itself though has disappeared. More commonly the collapse is partial and the characteristic appearance of the abnormal lobe as it collapses anteriorly and medially is shown in Fig. 3.29.

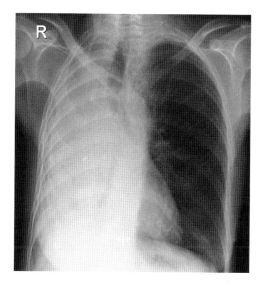

**Figure 3.28**
Complete collapse of the right lung in a lady who had carcinoma of the bronchus. The mediastinal shift is obvious, and the trachea is considerably deviated to the abnormal side.

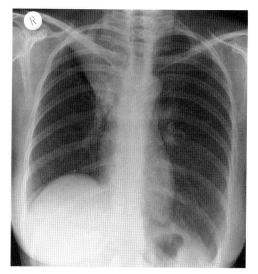

**Figure 3.29** Right upper lobe collapse. The abnormal lung is completely solid.

## Left upper lobe

The left upper lobe creates an unmistakeable pattern as it loses volume (shown classically in Fig. 3.30), and it rarely disappears completely. Note from Fig. 3.30 how the

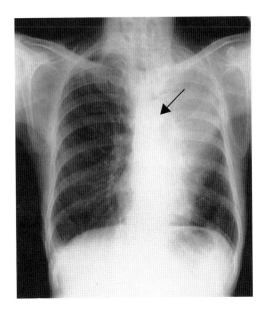

**Figure 3.30** Classical left upper lobe collapse.

consolidated lobe becomes progressively less dense from top to bottom. This is simply a reflection of the depth of lung tissue contained within it at different levels. Note also the hallmark 'comma' of aerated lung outlining the aortic knuckle (arrowed on Figs 3.30 and 3.32). This is probably derived from normal right lung herniating across the mid-line, which is, in itself, a fairly dramatic example of 'shift of normal structures'. Figure 3.32 is a subtler example and Fig. 3.31 is the lateral view of Fig. 3.30, included to illustrate the predominantly anterior movement of the left oblique fissure.

### Middle lobe

Figure 3.33 demonstrates a solid middle lobe with minimal loss of volume. In contrast, the minimal 'fuzziness' at the right heart border caused by complete middle lobe collapse (Fig. 3.35), so easy to overlook, emphasizes the need for a low threshold in suspecting middle lobe pathology on the postero-anterior (p–a) chest radiograph. (Just to prove that I am not cheating, Fig. 3.34 is the corresponding lateral view.)

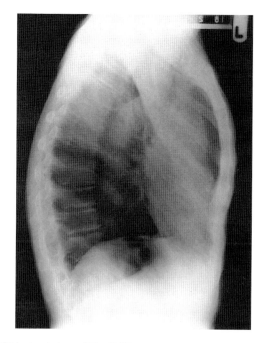

**Figure 3.31** Lateral view of Fig. 3.30.

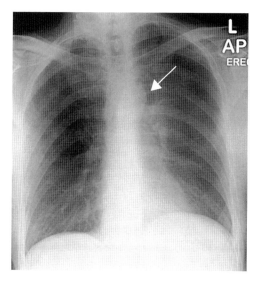

**Figure 3.32** Left upper lobe collapse with shift of the hemidiaphragm. Note the 'comma' of aerated lung (arrowed) as mentioned in the text.

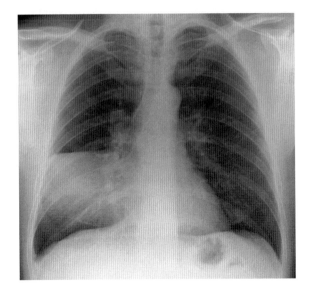

**Figure 3.33** Middle lobe consolidation and partial collapse (underlying tumour).

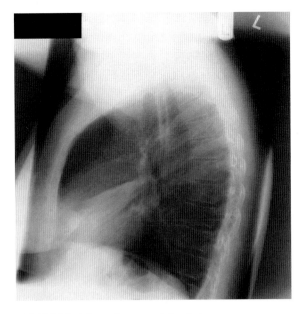

**Figure 3.34** Middle lobe collapse on lateral view.

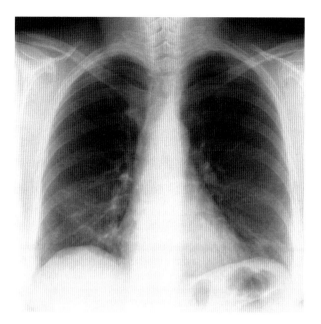

**Figure 3.35** Postero-anterior view of Fig. 3.34. The abnormality is minimal, manifest merely as blurring of the right heart border.

*Lingula*

Complete collapse of the lingula is even less striking on p–a view (Figs 3.36 and 3.37).

*Right lower lobe*

Figure 3.38 is an example of complete collapse of the right lower lobe. The characteristic 'sail-shape' shadow is obvious and the downward shift of the right hilum is marked. In addition, the right paravertebral structures and the medial right hemidiaphragm are both obscured by adjacent solid lung.

*Left lower lobe*

Figure 3.26 (page 74) is a classical example of left lower lobe collapse, demonstrating each of the three fundamental categories of radiographic signs of collapse. Figure 3.39 is a little more subtle, probably because the degree of collapse is

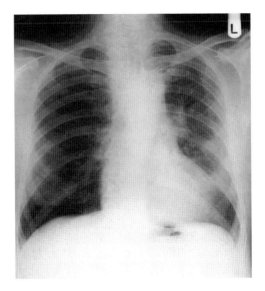

**Figure 3.36** Collapse of lingula: postero-anterior view.

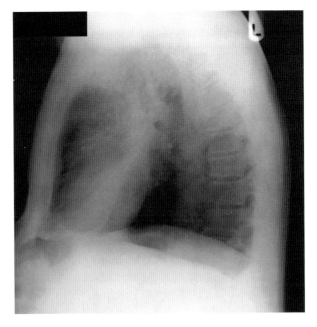

**Figure 3.37** Collapse of lingula: lateral view.

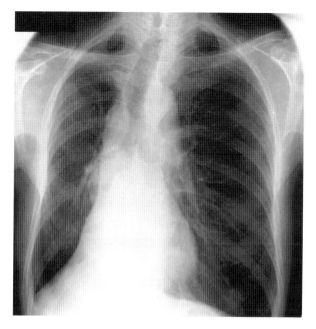

**Figure 3.38** Right lower lobe collapse.

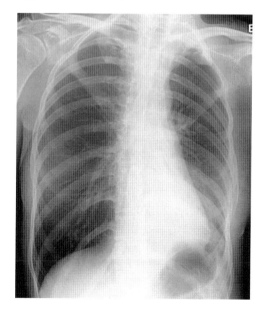

**Figure 3.39** Left lower lobe collapse.

not quite so marked. Nevertheless, the left hilum has nearly disappeared behind the heart shadow, the left hemidiaphragm and paravertebral shadow are obscured and the upward shift of the diaphragm can be inferred from the position of the stomach air bubble.

## CAVITATION

Put simply, the radiographic appearance of cavitation is created by destruction of tissue within existing abnormal areas of lung. It follows that cavities usually have thick-walled boundaries and this serves to distinguish them from conditions causing thin-walled ring shadows. These are covered in the next chapter.

Many different pathological processes in the lung can result in cavitation and we have seen a number of examples already (Figs 3.17–3.20, pages 68 and 69).

 **CLINICAL CONSIDERATIONS**

When pneumonic consolidation cavitates, this offers clues as to the potential infecting organism. Cavitating pneumonias are generically very unpleasant from a clinical point of view.

To complete this chapter, I have listed some examples of other causes of cavitation. They provide the opportunity to describe the specific radiographic features with which each is associated.

### Tuberculosis

Post-primary infection is the variety of tuberculosis that typically cavitates although, occasionally, primary foci of infection can progress in this way (Fig. 3.18, page 68). Post-primary disease tends to affect the apical and posterior parts of the lungs and both upper and lower lobes may be involved in this way.

**PEARL OF WISDOM**

This anatomical distribution is explained simply by the ventilation–perfusion relationship of different parts of the lungs. Mycobacteria like to be ventilated but not perfused – conditions pertaining in the apical area of each major lobe. This preference is further illustrated in bats, animals that spend a large part of their life hanging upside-down – they have foci of mycobacterial infection at their lung bases! It also explains why various pre-antibiotic era, surgical treatments for tuberculosis were successful. They were all based on the principle of 'resting' infected areas of lung, reducing the degree of ventilation within them.

Post-primary tuberculous infection is usually associated with considerable fibrosis and these factors conspire to produce a radiographic picture that is quite typical with bilateral upper zone fibrosis, shrinkage and cavitation (Fig. 3.40). Other conditions can mimic these appearances, however, and they are discussed in the following chapter.

## Aspergilloma

The fungus-ball of *Aspergillus*, also known as a mycetoma, is an opportunist development. The fungus traditionally grows in old tuberculous cavities but can in fact colonize any area of devitalized lung. There are well-documented examples in cavities caused by chronic sarcoidosis and in those associated with ankylosing spondylitis.

**CLINICAL CONSIDERATIONS**

In the days when tuberculosis was common it was well recognized that aspergillus did not colonize active tuberculous cavities; the fungus and the mycobacterium do not flourish together.

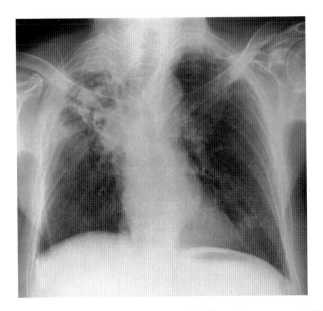

**Figure 3.40** Reactivation of tuberculosis with bilateral upper zone infiltration and shrinkage and apical pleural thickening. Cavitation can be clearly seen on the right.

The typical radiographic appearances of aspergilloma are those of a cavity filled with a round shadow that represents the fungus ball. This creates the classical 'halo sign' that is illustrated and arrowed in Fig. 3.41. Continued fungus growth may be accompanied by progressive apical pleural thickening over the surface of the colonized cavity. Indeed, sometimes this progressive pleural change is far more impressive than the size of the fungus ball itself.

## Primary lung abscess

Primary lung abscess is not common in these days of powerful antibiotics. When it does occur it may be associated with malignant proximal bronchial obstruction or with alcohol abuse and poor dental hygiene. This is described in the lower social classes in South Africa where, presumably, aspiration is the linking factor. Unusual organisms can be

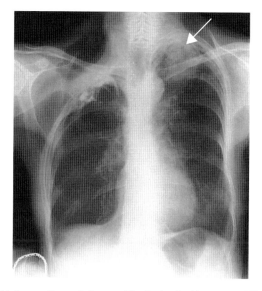

**Figure 3.41** Aspergilloma left apex. The 'halo sign' is arrowed. This merely reflects the presence of the fungus ball within a cavity. Note also the evidence of previous right thoracoplasty and the typical pattern of pleural calcification within an old tuberculous empyema at the right apex.

responsible for abscess formation and these include the filamentous bacterium, *Actinomyces*. The example illustrated in Fig. 3.20 (page 69) was actually caused by gonococcal infection, the source of which was never identified.

## Multiple lung abscesses

Figure 3.42 shows multiple lung abscesses, blood-borne from primary pelvic infection. There is obvious cavitation within the largest lesion.

Figure 3.43 is the X-ray of a man who suffered devastating staphylococcal pneumonia following influenza. Amazingly, he survived and his X-ray some years after the acute illness shows scattered micronodular calcification. It is featured in the next chapter.

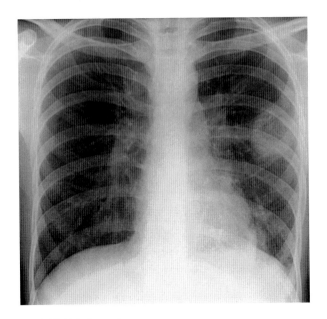

**Figure 3.42** Multiple lung abscesses.

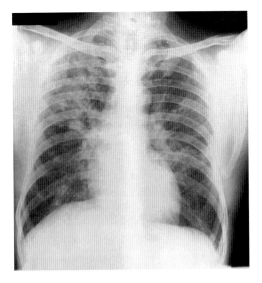

**Figure 3.43** Staphylococcal pneumonia following influenza.

Figure 3.44 depicts aggressive tuberculosis in a lady who was immunocompromised by virtue of treatment for extensive carcinoma of the breast. She responded well to antibiotic therapy, but note the malignant deposits in the right ribs.

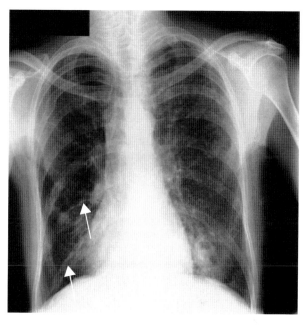

**Figure 3.44** Rapidly progressive tuberculosis in a lady receiving chemotherapy for carcinoma of the breast. Note the malignant deposits in several ribs (arrowed).

## Central necrosis

Central necrosis occurs in a number of other pathological processes. Pulmonary infarction is an example, so are rheumatoid nodules (Fig. 3.45) and progressive massive fibrosis, that is to say complicated coal-workers' pneumoconiosis (Fig. 3.46).

The next chapter continues the theme of describing patterns of abnormal intrapulmonary shadowing but concentrates on pulmonary infiltrations of various types as well as discussing cystic shadows and the causes of intrapulmonary calcification.

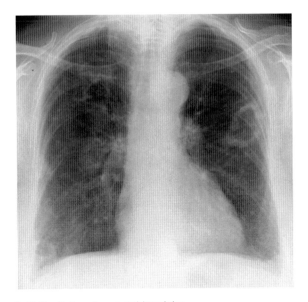

**Figure 3.45** Cavitating rheumatoid nodules.

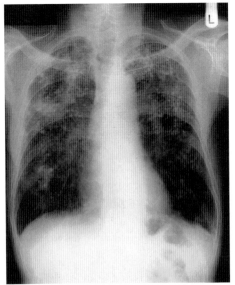

**Figure 3.46** This coal-worker had circulating rheumatoid factor. The calcified lesions in both lung fields are examples of the modified definition of Caplan's syndrome (Chapter 4, page 132). A coalescence of these nodules is shown and this has cavitated.

# PULMONARY INFILTRATES, NODULAR LESIONS, RING SHADOWS AND CALCIFICATION

The previous chapter examined the relationship between the radiographic pattern of alveolar filling and the pathological process of consolidation. It sought to describe an analytical process whereby pathological differential diagnosis might be narrowed by systematic investigation of details and variations in the basic radiographic pattern. The aim of this chapter is to construct a similar system for relating radiographic appearances to specific pathological aetiologies but instead of disease processes that result in alveolar filling we will consider a concatenation of clinical conditions that present as pulmonary infiltration, nodulation, large well-defined masses or calcification when they affect the lungs.

The diversity of abnormal intrapulmonary shadowing is superficially baffling and it represents an enormous differential diagnosis pathologically – something of a challenge. However, there is a systematic way to unravel the complexities and by engaging a few simple rules when examining an abnormal chest radiograph, the differential diagnosis can be narrowed to a few possibilities in the majority of cases and result in a firm diagnosis in a significant proportion of them.

This approach is based on two parallel assessments; the first addresses the morphology of the abnormal shadowing and the second concentrates on its distribution.

As with everything else in clinical medicine there are no absolutes in these definitions and there will certainly be exceptions to the lists of differential diagnoses constructed from this parallel approach. Nevertheless, the technique is useful because it is quick and practical and, most importantly, it is safe. This two-pronged approach to investigation should be combined with other basic observations:

- are the lung volumes maintained?
- is cardiomegaly present?
- are there associated pleural, bony or mediastinal shadows?
- are there other specific radiographic appearances that give the diagnosis away? An example here is the close association between septal lines and the pathological diagnoses of left heart failure or lymphangitis carcinomatosa.

## DEFINITION OF TERMS USED IN DESCRIBING ABNORMAL PULMONARY SHADOWING

It is essential to be absolutely clear about the meaning of the descriptive terms used. I think that it is best to describe exactly what you see and to avoid over-colourful terminology. Nevertheless, describing an abnormality as 'honeycombing', for example, is useful provided that there is a strict under-standing of what is meant by the terminology. In fact the pathological causes of true generalized honeycombing on a chest radiograph are few and it will be profitable to recognize and describe this pattern accurately.

The definitions that follow are fairly standard and, although the measurements quoted are inevitably arbitrary, they are based on years of confirmed practical usefulness. It is important to practise using these terms, to become comfortable with them and to be strict about avoiding vague descriptions that are open to interpretation.

## Circular shadows

These are best categorized according to size.

- **Micronodular shadows:** this is my preferred term and is better, I think, than the common synonyms, 'pinpoint' or 'fine mottling'. These rounded shadows are small, 1.5 mm or less in diameter.
- **Nodular shadows** are larger, up to 2 cm in diameter.
- **Large circular shadows** are 2 cm or more in diameter.

These shadows all have well-defined borders.

## Ill-defined shadows

This is a descriptive term for poorly defined shadows. They may be roughly circular or oval in shape ('blotchy' shadows) or have irregular boundaries, in which case their appearance merges with that of patchy consolidation.

## Linear shadows

These vary from 'hair-line' to 2 mm in thickness. Simon (see Further Reading list) describes wider band-like shadows as 'toothpaste' shadows and similar thickness linear shadows with bulbous ends as 'gloved finger' shadows (Fig. 4.1). I think these terms are useful because they are specific and both of them are most commonly seen in bronchiectasis, where they probably represent mucus-filled bronchi.

## Reticulo-nodular shadowing

This is used to describe a mix of linear and nodular shadowing in varying proportions. The nodular component is usually micronodular or small nodular in size.

## Small ring shadows, the honeycomb pattern

I have used this term to describe thin-walled ring shadows each enclosing a relatively radiolucent zone and each measuring up to about 1 cm in diameter.

## Larger ring shadows

Large ring shadows should be categorized according to their diameter and also with regard to the thickness of their boundary wall. Cavitation within an area of consolidation can manifest as a thick-walled ring shadow, and definitions can become blurred under these circumstances. Bronchogenic cysts and congenital parenchymal cysts present radiographically as large ring shadows with thin walls.

# TUBULAR SHADOWS

This term applies to two, more or less parallel, fine lines that enclose a radiolucent area (Fig. 4.1). The synonym, 'tram-line shadow' can be used when the shadow is the expected size of a bronchus and occurs in a position and

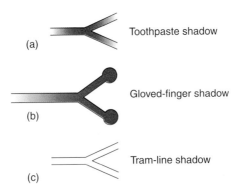

**Figure 4.1** Diagram to show 'toothpaste', 'gloved-finger' and 'tubular' shadows. After Simon (1978; see Further Reading list).

with the orientation that might be expected of a bronchus. When this applies the 'tram-line' represents a visible bronchus with thickened walls – again characteristically seen in bronchiectasis.

## Septal or interstitial lines (Fig. 2; page ix)

These are horizontal line shadows, usually 1–2 mm wide and commonly multiple. They are seen particularly above the costo-phrenic recesses and the lines most commonly measure 1.5–2 cm in length. As I have mentioned, this easily recognizable radiographic appearance is very helpful diagnostically, being particularly associated with left heart failure, lymphangitis carcinomatosa and coal-workers' pneumoconiosis. They are commonly known by the eponymous title, 'Kerley B lines' but I have preferred to use the descriptive terminology.

## DISTRIBUTION OF ABNORMAL SHADOWING

Once again, I emphasize that the descriptions that follow are intended only as a guide. There are common exceptions to the differential pathologies I have listed in association with each of the distribution patterns described. Moreover, grey areas abound as far as the distribution patterns themselves are concerned.

Another important point is that the radiographic appearances typical of a more acute stage of a disease process may be very different from the equally typical appearances that accompany the more chronic stages of the same disease. Sarcoidosis and extrinsic allergic alveolitis are two good examples of this, and visual examples of acute and chronic sarcoidosis are included in the illustrations that follow.

**CLINICAL CONSIDERATIONS**

The radiographic appearances of sarcoidosis have been usefully categorized into four stages:

- **Stage 1** refers to hilar and/or mediastinal lymphadenopathy in the absence of pulmonary infiltration
- **Stage 2** is the concurrent appearance of infiltration and lymphadenopathy
- **Stage 3** occurs when lymphadenopathy has disappeared but the infiltrate remains
- **Stage 4** is heralded by the advent of pulmonary fibrosis, usually manifest as upper zone shrinkage and increasing linear shadowing.

There are interesting epidemiological data from Sweden, which record the relative frequency of these radiographic stages.

The prevalence of presentation falls steadily from Stage 1 through to Stage 4.

Furthermore, the radiographic appearances of some disease processes are legion so it is almost pointless attempting to fit them into lists; leukaemic and lymphomatous infiltrates and drug-induced pulmonary infiltrates are typical examples.

Despite these qualifications, careful definition of the type of shadowing, and matching this to its radiographic distribution is a valuable exercise in determining the cause of widespread interstitial lung disease.

There are five schematic distribution patterns to consider and these are shown diagrammatically as reticulo-nodular infiltration in Fig. 4.2.

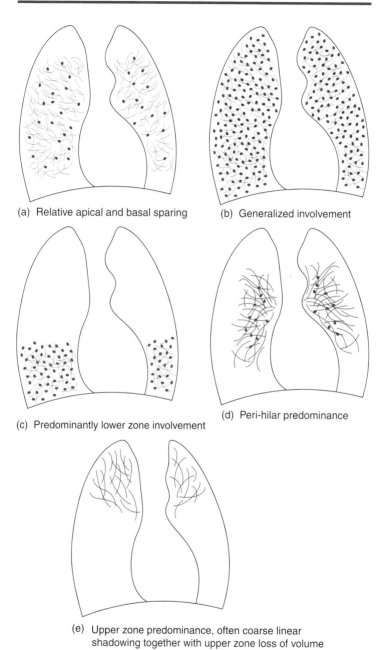

(a) Relative apical and basal sparing

(b) Generalized involvement

(c) Predominantly lower zone involvement

(d) Peri-hilar predominance

(e) Upper zone predominance, often coarse linear shadowing together with upper zone loss of volume

**Figure 4.2 (a–e)** Patterns of distribution of interstitial lung disease.

It is useful to consider these patterns in turn and in relation to the most likely pathological diagnoses that may be expected with each. I have additionally qualified the differential diagnosis in respect of the size of the nodular component that is predominant.

## Mid-zone distribution, with relative apical and basal sparing

● Micronodules or small nodules:
  ● sarcoidosis (Figs 4.3 and 4.4)
  ● coal-workers' pneumoconiosis (CWP; Fig. 4.5)
  ● *Pneumocystic carinii* infection (Fig. 4.6)

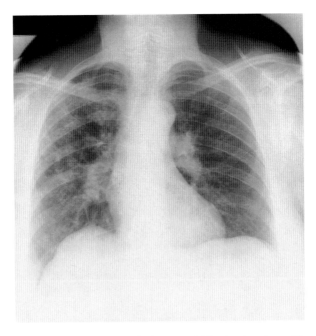

**Figure 4.3** Stage 2 sarcoidosis (pulmonary infiltration together with bilateral hilar lymphadenopathy). The infiltrate shows relative apical and basal sparing and the background nodulation is coalescing in areas.

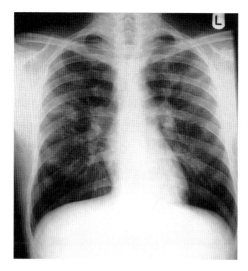

**Figure 4.4** Stage 2 sarcoidosis. In this example the mid-zone distribution of the infiltrate is still apparent in the left lung but the appearances are more widespread in the right.

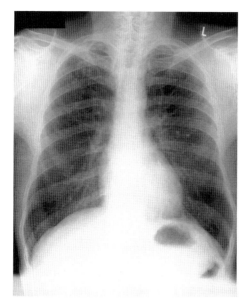

**Figure 4.5** Coal-workers' pneumoconiosis. The nodular infiltration in the mid-zones is subtle and this X-ray is a little unfair because there are slightly larger nodules in the upper zones. These were due to tuberculosis.

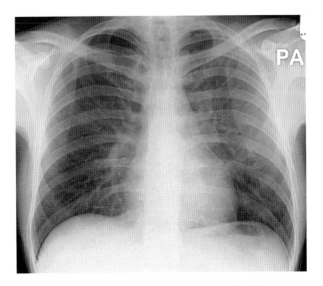

**Figure 4.6** *Pneumocystis carinii* pneumonia in acquired immune deficiency syndrome (AIDS) – there is shadowing predominantly in the mid-zones.

 **PEARL OF WISDOM**

Figure 4.5 is the X-ray of a man with simple CWP who developed pulmonary tuberculosis (PTB). This association was fortuitous, simple CWP does not predispose to PTB. In contrast, silicosis has a definite proclivity for predisposing to mycobacterial infection.

## All zones

- Micronodules:
    - miliary tuberculosis, (Figs 3.3, page 58, and 4.7).
      In Fig. 3.3, the background microdules can still be distinguished although their profusion resembles widespread consolidation at first sight.
    - CWP
    - sarcoidosis (rarely; Fig. 4.8).

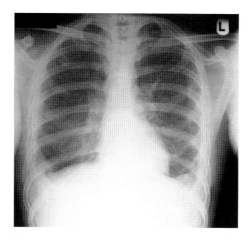

**Figure 4.7** Miliary tuberculosis. The micronodules are everywhere, even seen at the apices. This appearance and distribution is highly suggestive of tuberculosis.

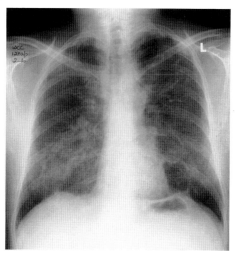

**Figure 4.8** This micronodular appearance of sarcoidosis is extremely rare and mimics miliary tuberculosis completely.

- Small nodules:
  - pneumonoconioses of various types including CWP (Fig. 4.9) and silicosis
  - pulmonary metastases, particularly from primary breast or thyroid malignancies (Fig. 4.10)

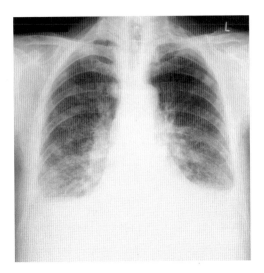

**Figure 4.9** Coal-workers' pneumocniosis. The background nodulation is due to coal-dust deposition. The bilateral pleural effusions appeared when this ex-miner developed nephrotic syndrome.

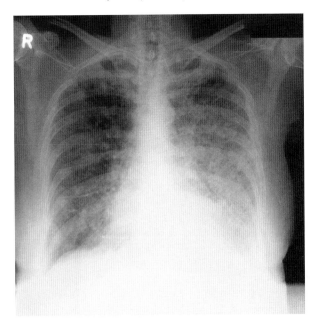

**Figure 4.10** These nodular metastases (some of them tiny) from a primary carcinoma of the breast are coalescing in several areas.

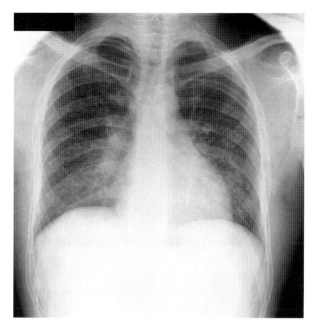

**Figure 4.11** Stage 2 sarcoidosis with widespread nodular pulmonary infiltration.

- sarcoidosis (Fig. 4.11),
- lymphangitis carcinomatosa (Fig. 4.12),
- extrinsic allergic alveolitis (acute; Fig. 4.13)
- drug induced (especially acute, e.g. methotrexate lung; Fig. 4.14)
- lymphoma (Fig. 4.15)
- haemosiderosis (acute)
- histoplasmosis (acute)
- pulmonary eosinophilia (Loeffler's syndrome and tropical eosinophilia)
- lymphangioleiomyomatosis/tuberose sclerosis (the infiltrate is a mix of nodules and micronodules and the appearance regularly progresses to manifest honeycombing; Fig. 4.16, page 106).
- Large nodules:
  - pulmonary metastases (Fig. 4.17, page 106).

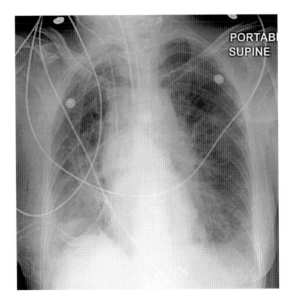

**Figure 4.12** This 64-year-old lady had lymphangitis carcinomatosa from a breast primary. The chest drain was required in order to deal with a large, malignant pleural effusion.

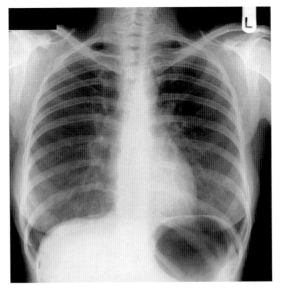

**Figure 4.13** Budgerigar-fanciers' lung. The widespread nodulation is subtle, the presenting symptoms were not.

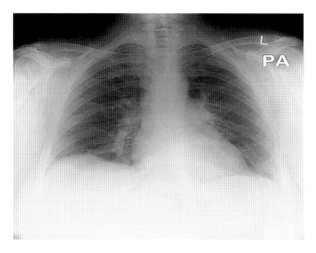

**Figure 4.14** Methotrexate-induced infiltration in a lady who had rheumatoid arthritis.

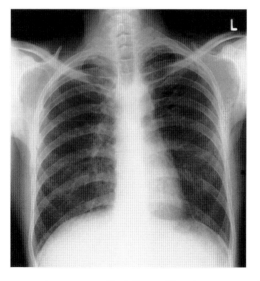

**Figure 4.15** The pulmonary manifestations of lymphoma are protean. In this case of Hodgkin's disease the pulmonary infiltrate is widespread and nodular in type.

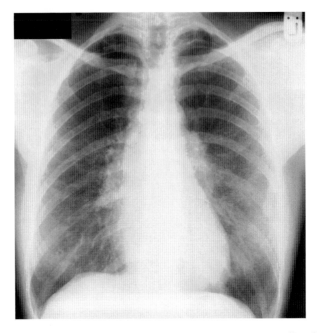

**Figure 4.16** Lymphangioleiomyomatosis. This young woman suffered progressive dyspnoea and had severe airways obstruction. The nodular (and micronodular) infiltrate can be seen and is, typically, in association with hyperexpanded lungs.

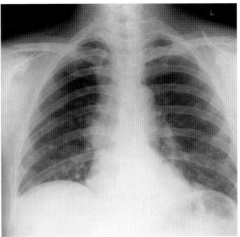

**Figure 4.17** Larger nodular metastases from a carcinoma of the bladder.

## CLINICAL CONSIDERATIONS

**Lymphangioleiomyomatosis.**   This rare condition is exclusive to women who are usually of child-bearing age. The pulmonary infiltration consists of extensive hamartomatous proliferation of smooth muscle in lung parenchyma and lymphatics, which also extends to surround small airways and pulmonary venules. In this way it is responsible for obstruction of lymphatics, small airways and blood vessels, and results in progressive airways obstruction. Pneumothorax is common and recurrent, and chylothorax is a well recognized complication as well.

There is evidence to suggest that the underlying cause is an imbalance between circulating or tissue oestrogen and progesterone levels and the number of tissue receptors for these hormones:

- the disorder has deteriorated during pregnancy
- progress of the disease slows after the menopause
- oophorectomy and/or progestogen treatment have benefited individual patients.

From a radiographic point of view the appearances are interesting because they manifest the unusual combination of a progressive pulmonary infiltration with lungs that are increasing in size rather than the opposite.

## Predominantly lower zones

- Micronodules:
  - haemosiderosis (chronic)
- Small nodules:
  - crytogenic fibrosing alveolitis (Figs 4.18–4.20),
  - rheumatoid fibrosing alveolitis

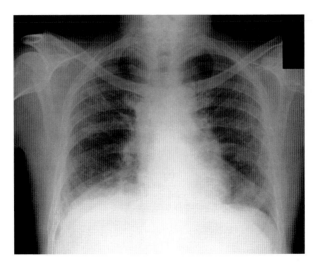

**Figure 4.18** Cryptogenic fibrosing alveolitis. Although the infiltration, which is often very linear, is predominantly lower zone in early stages, it then becomes more generalized as illustrated here. Nevertheless, the lower zone dominance is still apparent.

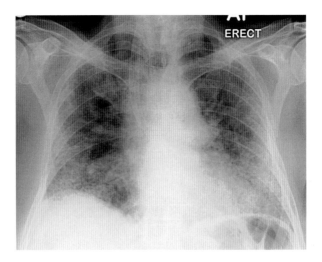

**Figure 4.19** This is advanced cryptogenic fibrosing alveolitis and dyspnoea was extreme. Note the small lungs, which had progressively shrunk as the disease inexorably progressed.

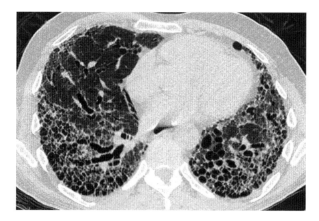

**Figure 4.20** The characteristic 'lace-work' pattern of the usual interstitial pneumonitis (UIP) type of cryptogenic fibrosing alveolitis. This is the CT scan of Fig. 4.19.

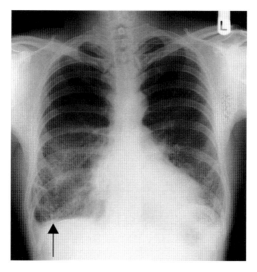

**Figure 4.21** Asbestosis. Obvious lower zone dominance of this reticulo-nodular infiltrate. There is localized honeycombing in the lower-right zone. Note the calcified plaque on the right hemidiaphragm (arrowed). Comprehensive examination of this radiograph secured the diagnosis.

- collagen vascular disease-associated fibrosing alveolitis
- asbestosis (Fig. 4.21).
- drug induced (especially chronic, e.g. bleomycin or busulphan lung).

## Peri-hilar distribution

- Nodules of varying sizes and often with confluent shadows as well
  - Left heart failure (Fig. 4.22)
  - adult respiratory distress syndrome (ARDS)
  - alveolar haemorrhage e.g. Goodpasture's syndrome (Fig. 4.23)
  - pulmonary alveolar proteinosis (Fig. 4.24)
  - lymphangitis carcinomatosa
  - *Pneumocystis carinii* pneumonia (PCP) (Fig. 4.25).

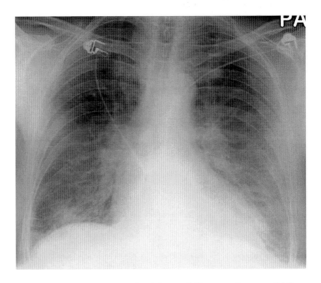

**Figure 4.22** Another example of left heart failure to show peri-hilar distribution. The background is quite nodular although it merges into an alveolar-filling pattern. Septal lines are clearly seen at the right base.

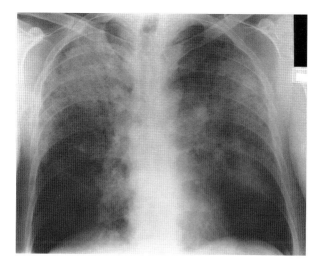

**Figure 4.23** Goodpasture's syndrome. This patient's haemoptysis was extreme but this isn't always the case.

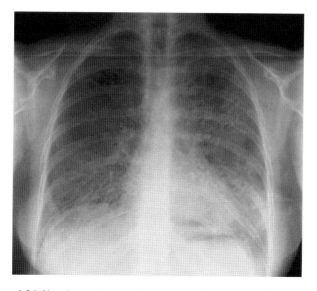

**Figure 4.24** Alveolar proteinosis. I have a number of examples of this condition, collected over the years, and these demonstrate its protean radiographic manifestations. This example started as peri-hilar distribution, but at the stage shown here, the appearances are more widespread and the nodular pattern is blurring into alveolar filling.

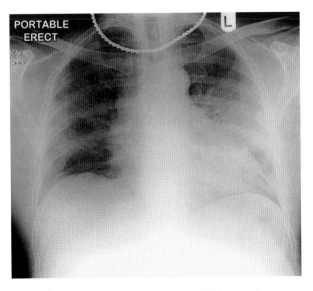

**Figure 4.25** *Pneumocystis carinii* pneumonia. Widespread reticulonodular infiltration in peri-hilar distribution. Once again nodules are merging into alveolar-filling.

**HAZARD**

Haemoptysis in alveolar haemorrhage may be minimal or even absent. This isn't the norm but it does happen, so consider the possibility, given appropriate radiographic change, even in the absence of visible blood clinically.

## Predominantly upper zones (with lung shrinkage and fibrosis if marked with an asterisk)

- Background of nodules of differing sizes:
  - sarcoidosis* (Fig. 4.26)
  - silicosis*
  - extrinsic allergic alveolitis (chronic)*
  - ankylosing spondylitis (mainly linear shadows)*
  - eosinophilic granuloma (early)
  - post-primary tuberculosis* (Fig. 3.40, page 86)
  - bronchopulmonary aspergillosis*

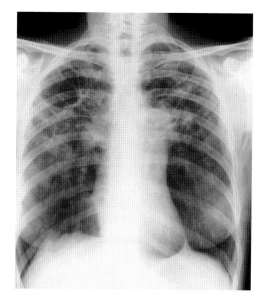

**Figure 4.26** Sarcoidosis with upper lobe fibrosis and shrinkage. Cavity formation is also apparent on the left. This appearance is equally compatible with the pulmonary changes of ankylosing spondylitis, silicosis and extrinsic allergic alveolitis, although gross cavitation is not typical of the latter.

- chronic *Klebsiella* pneumonia*
- complicated CWP, including progressive massive fibrosis and Caplan's syndrome (Fig. 4.27)
- rheumatoid nodules (Fig. 4.28).

## OTHER PATTERNS OF PULMONARY INFILTRATION

Fig. 4.29 shows three other patterns of pulmonary infiltration in diagrammatic form.

### Coarse large nodular pattern, often with blurred outline: 'blotchy shadowing'

- Bacterial pneumonia including tuberculosis (Fig. 4.30, page 116)
- Non-bacterial pneumonia e.g. Mycoplasma (Fig. 4.31, page 116)
- Viral pneumonia (Fig. 4.32, page 117).

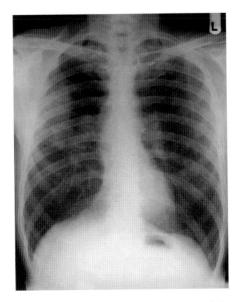

**Figure 4.27** Caplan's syndrome. Caplan nodules up to 1.5 cm in diameter are present in the upper zones and these have coalesced on the left. The background dust infiltration is minimal but septal lines are present at the left base.

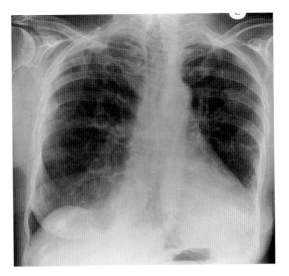

**Figure 4.28** Rheumatoid nodules.

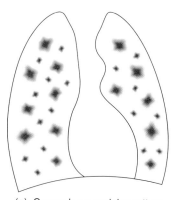

(a) Coarse large nodular pattern, often with blurred outlines

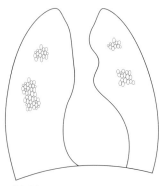

(b) 'Honeycombing'

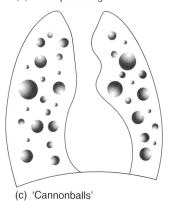

(c) 'Cannonballs'

**Figure 4.29 (a–c)** Three other patterns of intrapulmonary shadowing.

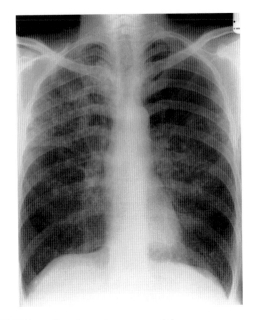

**Figure 4.30** 'Tuberculous bronchopneumonia'.

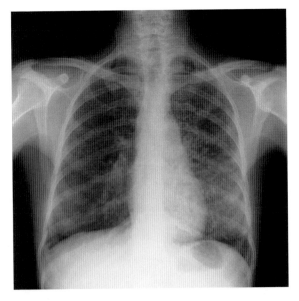

**Figure 4.31** Mycoplasma pneumonia.

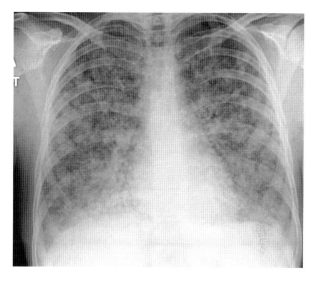

**Figure 4.32** Extensive chickenpox pneumonia in a young woman.

 **CLINICAL CONSIDERATIONS**

**Non-bacterial pneumonia.** The radiographic appearances of *Mycoplasma* pneumonia vary from typical lobar consolidation to the pattern just illustrated. What is often striking clinically is that the physical signs are unimpressive even though the radiographic changes may be dramatic.

The example of chickenpox pneumonia I have included is extreme. Lung involvement is more pronounced in older individuals with chickenpox and in those who are immunocompromised. The extent of pneumonic change also seems to be proportional to the severity of the skin rash, particularly in adults, and a profuse rash is a useful predictor of pulmonary complications under these circumstances.

- Cystic fibrosis (Fig. 4.33)
- Cryptogenic organizing pneumonitis (Fig. 4.34)
- PCP
- Fungal infection
- Malignant metastases (Fig. 4.35)
- Lung abscesses
- Vasculitis
- Pulmonary lymphoma (Fig. 4.36)
- Drug induced (Fig. 4.37)

I have included several illustrations and several pathologies in order to provide a flavour of the variability of 'blotchy' shadowing. You will see that the distinction between it and patchy consolidation can be difficult but then, realistically, with many disease processes, one might expect these appearances to merge one into the other anyway.

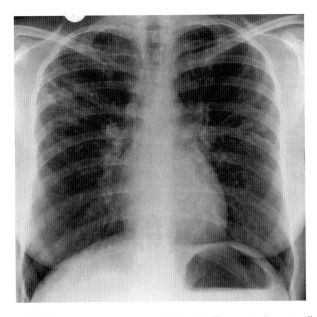

**Figure 4.33** This young lady has cystic fibrosis. The central venous line (for antibiotic administration) can be seen.

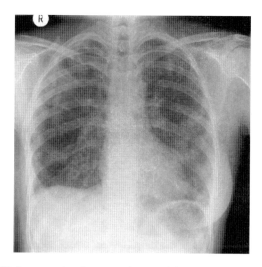

**Figure 4.34** An example of crytogenic organizing pneumonitis.

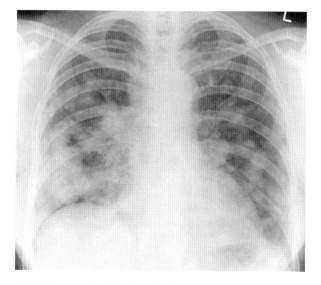

**Figure 4.35** These metastatic deposits from an endometrial carcinoma are not as well defined in outline as classical 'cannon-ball' secondaries.

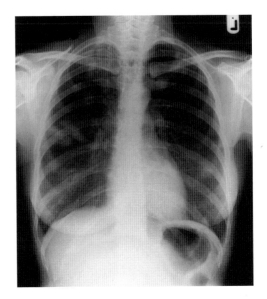

**Figure 4.36** This is the radiograph of a patient with an early pulmonary T-cell lymphoma.

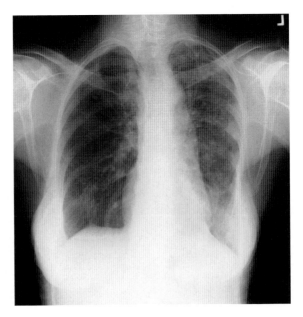

**Figure 4.37** 'Salazopyrine lung'.

## Honeycombing

This may be localized, in which case it is seen as a component in many pathological entities including sarcoidosis, fibrosing alveolitis, drug-induced lung disease (Fig. 4.38), extrinsic allergic alveolitis and lymphangitis carcinomatosa. When honeycombing is more extensive, the list of possibilities becomes smaller and includes lymphangioleiomyomatosis, tuberose sclerosis and bronchiectasis – although in the last condition the ring shadows are often thicker-walled (Fig. 4.39).

The most extreme examples of 'honeycomb lung' are virtually diagnostic of eosinophilic granuloma, a variant of histiocytosis X (Figs 4.40 and 4.41).

Single or multiple, large cystic structures with thin walls may represent emphysematous bullae (Fig. 1.23, page 19) or congenital, bronchogenic or parenchymal cysts (Fig. 4.42).

## 'Cannon-balls'

This graphic description of multiple, well-defined rounded shadows of varying sizes, some of them very large, is

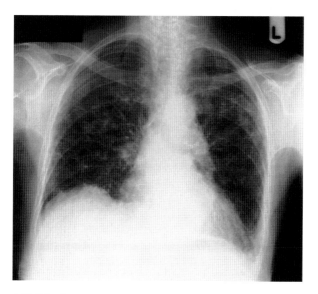

**Figure 4.38** 'Nitrofurantoin lung': to show localized honeycombing.

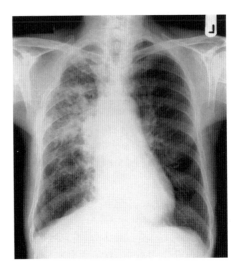

**Figure 4.39** Cystic bronchiectasis. This does show honeycombing but many of the ring shadows have rather thick walls. Also note the variability in diameter of the ring shadows and the right-sided predominance of the abnormality.

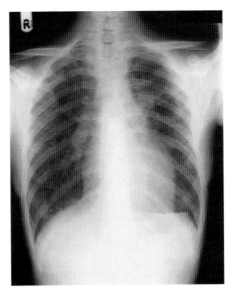

**Figure 4.40** Eosinophilic granuloma (histiocytosis X). Although honeycombing is present, a background nodular infiltrate can still be seen.

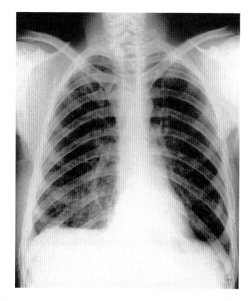

**Figure 4.41** Another example of eosinophilic granuloma. The pathology here is more advanced and this is manifest as classical honeycombing.

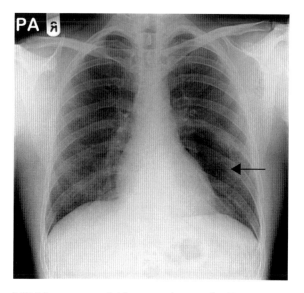

**Figure 4.42** A large congenital lung cyst (arrowed) adjacent to the left heart border.

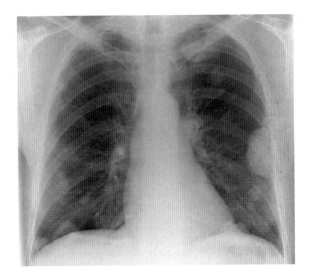

**Figure 4.43** Renal carcinoma metastases.

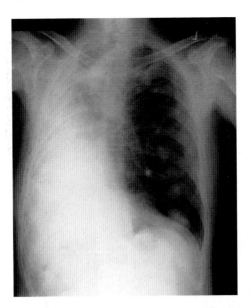

**Figure 4.44** 'Cannon-ball' metastases from a carcinoma of the bladder. This unfortunate man had undergone pneumonectomy for squamous cell carcinoma of the bronchus some years before these secondary deposits appeared.

reserved for malignant pulmonary metastases. Although they complicate a diverse selection of primary malignancies, 'cannon-balls' are traditionally associated with carcinomas of the genito-urinary tract. (Figs 4.43 and 4.44).

# THE SOLITARY PULMONARY NODULE

The boxed list gives a variety of clinical possibilities manifesting as a solitary intrapulmonary nodule on chest

## PATHOLOGICAL CAUSES OF A PULMONARY NODULE

- Bronchial carcinoma
- Metastasis*
- Granuloma (tuberculosis, sarcoidosis, vasculitis)* (Figs 4.45 and 4.46)
- Hamartoma
- Bronchial adenoma
- Lymphoma*
- Abscess*
- 'Round pneumonia' (Fig. 4.47)
- Rheumatoid nodule*
- Round atelectasis (Figs 4.48 and 4.49, page 128)
- Pneumoconiosis (progressive massive fibrosis, Caplan's syndrome)*
- Arteriovenous malformation
- Pulmonary infarct*
- Haematoma
- Fluid-filled cyst or bulla

Notes: an asterisk indicates that these conditions usually cause multiple lesions. The list is not exhaustive; it indicates the commoner possibilities that should be considered in your differential diagnosis.

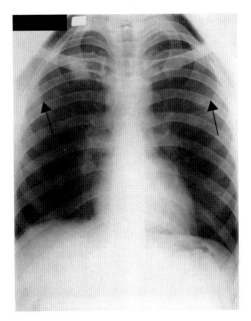

**Figure 4.45** Sarcoidosis. The nodule in the right upper zone is clearly seen but close scrutiny will show other faint opacities, arrowed, on both sides.

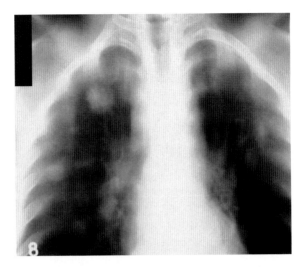

**Figure 4.46** The nodules in Fig. 4.45 are beautifully shown here on old-fashioned tomography. This is a most unusual appearance for sarcoidosis.

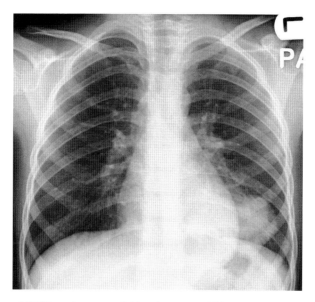

**Figure 4.47** 'Round pneumonia' in a four-year-old boy.

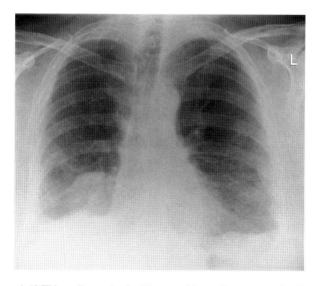

**Figure 4.48** This radiograph of a 79-year-old man is an example of round atelectasis. He had a history of significant asbestos exposure.

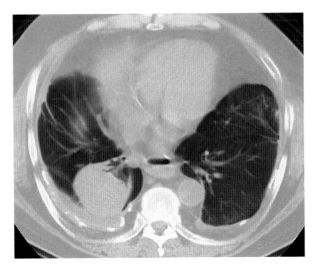

**Figure 4.49** This is a CT image of the same lesion as in Fig. 4.48 showing it to be contiguous with a pleural plaque. This man had worked with asbestos.

radiograph. The differential diagnosis can be honed through classical radiological detective work, although the definitive diagnosis will often require additional imaging techniques and quite probably a biopsy procedure as well.

 **CLINICAL CONSIDERATIONS**

**Round pneumonia and round atelectasis.**   Round pneumonia probably represents an early stage of what will develop into lobar pneumonic consolidation. It is interesting that this appearance is especially seen in children and also that it is now being reported in cases of severe acute respiratory syndrome (SARS).

Round atelectasis is probably caused by infolding of the pleura and is well-recognized in association with asbestos-induced pleural disease.

A reasonable approach to radiographic interpretation of the solitary pulmonary nodule is as follows:

1 **Is its margin well-defined?**
   Malignancies tend to be well defined, though not always and not exclusively so either. A pulmonary infarction, for instance, can be very well circumscribed and I have shown examples of round pneumonia and round atelectasis, neither of them malignant in pathology.

**PEARL OF WISDOM**

**Particular appearances of malignancy.** Occasionally, the border of a pulmonary nodule has an irregular, spiculated or 'thorny' appearance. This has been called the 'corona maligna' (malignant crown) and the appearance should make you suspicious of malignant disease although granulomata are well documented as producing a similar appearance.

2 **Has the nodule changed in size rapidly?**
   Rapid growth usually indicates malignancy but, on the other hand, some carcinomas can be very slow growing.
3 **Does the nodule contain calcium?**
   In the UK, most calcified nodules are tuberculous in origin. Histoplasmosis is a common cause in endemic areas and it may produce a characteristic 'bull's-eye' appearance with calcium at the centre of the nodule.

**HAZARD**

Although calcification is highly suggestive of benignity, a granuloma can become complicated by a pulmonary malignancy, the so-called 'scar cancer', so beware.

More reassuring is the scattered, intralesional, 'popcorn' calcification displayed by some hamartomas (Fig. 4.50).

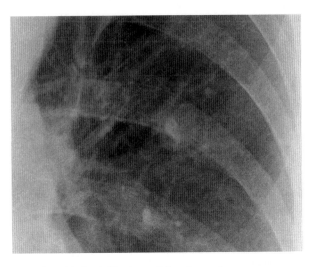

**Figure 4.50** Speckled calcification within a hamartoma.

4   Is the lesion accompanied by significant collapse?
    Localized segmental or lobar collapse is suggestive of
    malignancy as we have already discussed.
5   Is there associated pleural, bony or lymph node disease?
    All of these features ring alarm bells that the pathology
    may be malignant (Fig. 4.51).

## DIFFUSE INTRAPULMONARY CALCIFICATION

Diffuse pulmonary calcinosis and diffuse pulmonary
ossification are generic terms describing the widespread
deposition of calcium and bone, respectively, in the lung
parenchyma.

● Pulmonary calcinosis is recognized in hyperparathy-
  roidism, chronic renal disease, vitamin D intoxification, very
  occasionally in pseudoxanthoma elasticum and also in association with malignant tumours causing hypercalcaemia.
● Pulmonary ossification is usually idiopathic but was hitherto associated with chronic mitral stenosis and can complicate amyloidosis.

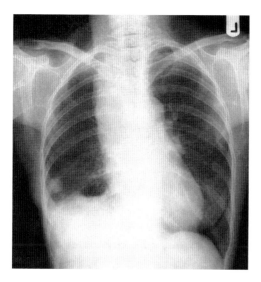

**Figure 4.51** An intrapulmonary nodule accompanied by extensive mediastinal lymphadenopathy and an ipsilateral pleural effusion. Unfortunately, the expected diagnosis of oat-cell carcinoma was confirmed.

Both conditions are vanishingly rare but there are other causes of intrapulmonary calcification that we do see, and differentiating these is relatively straightforward – most of the time!

● **Old healed pulmonary tuberculosis.** The calcification may be micronodular or, more commonly, the nodules are between 2 and 10 mm in diameter. They may be widespread and, in the case of the miliary (micronodular) pattern can be identified right into the lung apices. Look for associated pleural changes.
● **Previous chickenpox.** The calcified lesions are usually micronodular and not so profuse. They merely represent healed viral pneumonic change (Fig. 4.52).
● **Industrial lung disease.** Not many of the pneumoconioses calcify. The exceptions are:
  ● **silicosis:** silica (unlike coal dust) is highly fibrogenic and its early, predominantly mid-zone deposition is readily accompanied by upper zone shrinkage. So look for loss of volume as well as accompanying 'egg-shell' calcification of the hilar lymph nodes.

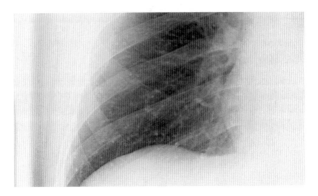

**Figure 4.52** Detail of right lower lobe showing micronodular calcification due to previous chickenpox pneumonia.

- Caplan's syndrome: this form of progressive massive fibrosis is allowed to evolve when the inhaled insult of coal-dust is accompanied by the presence of circulating rheumatoid factor (Fig. 4.27, page 114).

 **PEARL OF WISDOM**

Caplan was a radiologist in Cardiff, who, in the 1950s, described the syndrome that bears his name when he noticed an association between progressive massive fibrosis (PMF) and circulating rheumatoid factor. There were two observations that made the miners he described remarkable. The first was the paucity of their background simple pneumoconiosis (usually in PMF the background nodulation is heavy, reflecting the dust load in the lungs) and the second was the presence of (often mild) rheumatoid arthritis. It later became clear that arthritis did not have to be present but rheumatoid factor did. Pathologically, it seems that there is some synergistic interplay between rheumatoid factor and coal-dust in initiating this type of lung injury. Caplan also noticed that this variety of PMF had a proclivity to calcify whereas 'normal' PMF didn't. Caplan's original description was of large areas of fibrosis but the story was completed a few years later when he described his 'extended definition' of the syndrome where the nodules were more numerous and smaller, several millimetres to several centimetres in diameter. This is the variety shown in Fig. 4.27. Altogether, of course, this is a marvellous story of the combination of astute radiological observation and brilliant clinical detective work.

- Other radio-dense but non-calcific pneumoconioses include stannosis, siderosis, baritosis and talc-workers' lung.

 **CLINICAL CONSIDERATIONS**

Interestingly, the radiographic appearances of barium and iron diminish if exposure ceases, and this is due to effective mechanisms of clearance of the dusts. This is certainly not the case with silica, which can progress (and calcify) after exposure has ended.

- Fungal infections:
  - **histoplasmosis**: the major endemic areas for this infection are the great river valleys of North America.
  - **coccidioidomycosis** can also result in diffuse pulmonary calcification. It is caused by inhalation of a soil-living fungus that thrives in semi-arid conditions. It is endemic from 40 degrees North, 120 degrees West in California to 40 degrees South, 65 degrees West in Argentina.
- Rarities:
  - **osteogenic sarcoma**: secondary deposits are reported to have been responsible for diffuse intrapulmonary calcification, but the likelihood of a patient surviving with such an aggressive primary malignancy for sufficient time to allow the radiographic changes to develop is remote.
  - **calcification following staphylococcal pneumonia**: this really does occur, though rarely. It is not known whether

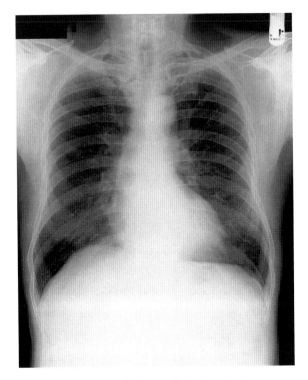

**Figure 4.53** Intrapulmonary calcification following staphylococcal pneumonia.

    it is a phenomenon precipitated by the *Staphylococcus* or the viral pneumonia, which may have preceded the bacterial infection (Fig. 4.53).

- **pulmonary alveolar microlithiasis**: in this condition of unknown cause, calcified, 'onion-skin' spherical structures are found within alveoli. These lesions can eventually ossify and there is a striking discrepancy in the lack of clinical symptoms compared with the apparently horrific radiographic findings.

This completes the discussion on pulmonary infiltrates and other abnormal patterns of intrapulmonary shadowing. In the next chapter we concentrate on the radiographic appearances of pleural disease.

# 5

# PLEURAL DISEASE

The large number of disease processes that affect the lung parenchyma, and the diversity of the intrapulmonary shadowing that they cause have been the subjects of the previous two chapters. Many diseases involve and invade the pleura as well, but when they do so, the variety of radiographic shadowing that results is limited. Basically, this chapter is concerned with a description of the radiographic appearances that result from the presence of air (pneumothorax), fluid (pleural effusion), pus (empyema) and solid tumour (primary and secondary) within the pleural cavity. Just to make life interesting there are combinations of these 'fillings' (hydropneumothorax, pyopneumothorax and so on) and pleural fluid may be composed of transudate or exudate, blood or, rarely, chyle. There are characteristic patterns of pleural calcification also and it is with a discussion of these that the chapter ends.

The management of pleural disease is not always easy. There are serious potential diagnostic pitfalls and accurate radiographic interpretation is paramount in avoiding these. Clinical management and radiographic diagnosis are intimately interwoven when dealing with pleural disease and this interplay provides much of the emphasis of this chapter. Please note the 'Hazard' boxes. These mistakes are regularly perpetrated, sometimes with severe clinical consequences.

## PNEUMOTHORAX (Fig. 1.22, page 19)

Just a little physiology to start! It does help in understanding the management and prognosis of this condition.

Intra-alveolar pressure is greater than intrapleural pressure. It follows that if an alveolus ruptures air will pass into the pleural space until the pressure equalizes. The pressure changes that occur within the affected hemithorax result in depression of the hemidiaphragm and shift of the mediastinum to the opposite side. If the degree of mediastinal shift is sufficient to compromise the normal lung and to affect venous return (and therefore cardiac output) the pneumothorax is said to be under 'tension'. This is a medical emergency, the radiographic hallmark of which is significant mediastinal shift and the clinical hallmark, tracheal deviation on palpation in the suprasternal notch.

 **HAZARD**

Even relatively small pneumothoraces can result in tension, the reason probably being that the visceral pleura creates a flap over the leak and operates as a ball-valve, allowing air to pass into the pleural space on inspiration, but preventing its escape during expiration. A dramatic increase in intrapleural pressure can subsequently occur, sometimes with relatively small volume change. **Always check clinically and radiographically for mediastinal shift.**

 **CLINICAL CONSIDERATIONS**

Once the air leak seals and accumulation of the pneumothorax ceases, re-expansion will take place at the rate of 1.25 per cent of the volume of the hemithorax per day. This natural reabsorption is speeded by administering oxygen.

Pneumothoraces are either spontaneous or traumatic, and spontaneous pneumothoraces can be primary or secondary depending on the presence or absence of underlying lung disease. Primary spontaneous pneumothorax is a common condition particularly in young men, the male:female ratio is 3:1. It results from rupture of a surface bleb towards the apex of the lung. Tall people are particularly prone to developing such blebs because in them the distance from the apex to the base of the lung is greater and there is therefore more negative intrapleural pressure at their lung apices than in shorter people.

A number of conditions predispose to secondary spontaneous pneumothorax. These include, commonly, emphysema and asthma but also tuberculosis, sarcoidosis, cystic fibrosis and staphylococcal pneumonia (probably as a result of its propensity to cavitate). Uncommon pathologies that are complicated by recurrent pneumothoraces are histiocytosis X, pulmonary neurofibromatosis, lymphangioleiomyomatosis, Ehlers–Danlos and Marfan's syndromes and congenital lung cysts. The man with eosinophilic granuloma depicted in Fig. 4.41 (page 123) and the man with a lung cyst shown in Fig. 4.42 (page 123) both suffered pneumothoraces; this was a recurrent problem in the first case.

 **CLINICAL CONSIDERATIONS**

The physiological effects of a pneumothorax are exaggerated in the presence of underlying lung disease as indeed are the symptoms that the patient experiences. The corollary to this statement is that the threshold for inserting an intercostal drain is lower in those with underlying lung disease.

A small primary spontaneous pneumothorax probably requires no treatment. The problem rests in defining what is meant by 'small', the traditional defintion being 'less than 20 per cent in volume of the hemithorax'. I would counsel more flexibility in this judgement depending on symptoms, length of the history (if a lung is collapsed for a period of time its visceral pleura becomes thickened and less compliant to lung re-expansion) and, certainly, the presence of background lung disease.

## PEARL OF WISDOM

**Catamenial pneumothorax.** This condition is associated with intrapleural endometriosis; fragments of endometrial tissue probably find their way into the pleural space through diaphragmatic defects. The fact that such defects are commoner in the right hemidiaphragm explains why almost all documented cases of catamenial pneumothorax have been right-sided. At the onset of menstruation, the endometrial patch breaks down and a pneumothorax results. Always consider this diagnostic possibility in young women with recurrent pneumothoraces. The appropriate history will make the diagnosis – and your reputation!

The radiographic appearances do not, of course, help in distinguishing the cause of a pneumothorax unless there is evidence of underlying lung disease. There is little difficulty in recognizing a pneumothorax in the classical case with a rim of air surrounding a partially collapsed lung (Fig. 1.22, page 19), but you may have to concentrate to ensure identifying a small air leak. The challenge comes when the appearances are not typical, with localized or unusual accumulation of air perhaps because of pre-existing pleural adhesions.

## HAZARD

In particular, be absolutely sure that the air resides within the pleural space, and that the appearances are not caused by a bulla or a lung cyst. An intercostal drain inserted into a bulla or a cyst is not a good idea.

# PLEURAL EFFUSION

Table 5.1 provides a useful list of causes of pleural effusion, categorized according to prevalence and on the basis of their being either a transudate or an exudate.

**Table 5.1** Causes of pleural effusion

|  | **Common** | **Less common** |
|---|---|---|
| Transudates | Heart failure<br>Cirrhosis of the liver<br>Nephrotic syndrome | Myxoedema<br>Sarcoidosis<br>Peritoneal dialysis |
| Exudates |  |  |
|   Infection | Bacterial pneumonia<br>Tuberculosis<br>Subphrenic abscess | Viral pneumonia<br>Parasitic<br>  pneumonia |
|   Malignancy | Carcinoma of the<br>  bronchus<br>Secondary malignancy | Mesothelioma |
|   Collagen vascular | Rheumatoid arthritis<br>Systemic lupus<br>  erythematosus |  |
|   Pulmonary embolism |  |  |
|   Subdiaphragmatic<br>  causes | Subphrenic abscess | Pancreatitis<br>(virtually always<br>left-sided because<br>of the anatomical<br>relations of the<br>lesser sac) |
|   Trauma | Haemothorax | Chylothorax |

It is worthwhile considering other rare causes of pleural effusion which are described in the following list.

● **Benign asbestos pleurisy:** despite being well documented, this diagnosis is often missed. The effusions can be recurrent, and progressive pleural thickening can supervene with accompanying progressive breathlessness. This condition carries a risk of mesothelioma development but there is no evidence that this risk is greater than in individuals who have similar asbestos exposure but who do not have benign pleural disease.

● **Dressler's syndrome:** this was described originally as a late complication of cardiac surgery. It then became clear that an exactly similar syndrome followed myocardial infarction, and these days similar symptoms are probably commonest 6–12 weeks after coronary artery bypass grafting. Pericardial pain and fluid occur as well as pleurisy and the erythrocyte sedimentation rate (ESR) is often very elevated.

● **Familial Mediterranean fever:** ethnic background (Sephardic and Iraqui Jews, Arabs, Armenians and Turks) and an awareness of this possibility should ensure the diagnosis. The effusions are usually small and the main symptoms are abdominal pain and fever.

● **Meig's syndrome:** this describes ascites and pleural effusion in association with a fibroma of the ovary. Ascitic fluid tracks through diaphragmatic defects and the (potentially massive) effusion is therefore more commonly right-sided. Removal of the tumour removes the problem – this is a non-malignant condition.

● **Yellow nail syndrome:** the underlying problem in this condition is hypoplasia of lymphatic vessels, and the clinical manifestations as a result are deformed yellow nails, lymphoedema in the limbs, pleural effusions, which can be bilateral and sometimes massive, and occasionally bronchiectasis. The main clinical features of the syndrome may develop at widely different times, adding to the challenge of the diagnosis. When effusions are present though, the nails are usually abnormal.

## Radiographic appearances

The classical, radiographic appearance of a pleural effusion is unmistakeable – dependent fluid with a lateral meniscus as it tracks up the chest wall (Figs 4.51, page 131, and 5.1).

Sometimes, however, it can be difficult to differentiate fluid from pleural thickening and quite often it is tricky to decide where the hemidiaphragm lies on the affected side, an important

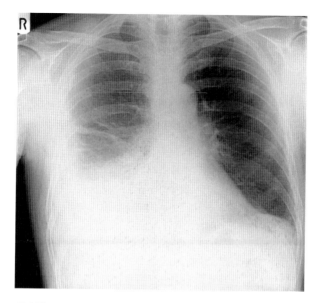

**Figure 5.1** Rheumatoid disease was responsible for this moderate-sized pleural effusion. There is also a widespread nodular pulmonary infiltrate caused by methotrexate. The infiltrate responded very well to corticosteroids.

decision if aspiration and/or biopsy is contemplated. Subpulmonary collections of fluid (Fig. 5.2), interlobar effusions and loculated fluid also demand special care and this is where ultrasound examination comes into its own.

In the patient depicted in Fig. 5.2, a right lateral decubitus radiograph confirmed the presence of fluid with a characteristic rim of fluid lying against the dependent right chest wall.

## HAZARD

Before aspirating or biopsying the pleural space be absolutely clear of the position of the diaphragm. If you don't know, seek experienced help. A needle in the liver or spleen may have dire consequences, particularly if it is an Abram's biopsy needle.

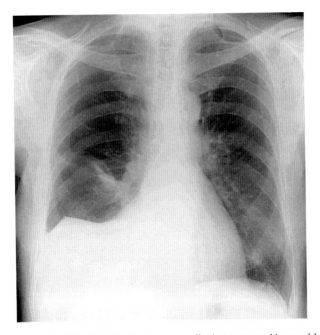

**Figure 5.2** This right-sided subpulmonary effusion occurred in an elderly man. Note the fluid in the lesser fissure also.

## Size of the effusion

Generally speaking, a large collection of fluid (let's say more than 50 per cent of the hemithorax) is highly suspicious of primary or secondary lung malignancy, mesothelioma or empyema. Having said that, rheumatoid effusions can be large, and, on occasion so can pneumonic effusions and those secondary to pulmonary embolism. With these qualifications in mind, however, the size of the effusion is helpful in arriving at the diagnosis.

Also informative in narrowing the differential diagnosis is the presence of pain. Embolic pleurisy is very painful, so is pleurisy associated with systemic lupus erythematosus, and if an effusion develops in either case it is usually small (in contrast, rheumatoid effusions are usually painless). Pleurisy occurring with pneumococcal pneumonia is another example of painful accumulation of pleural fluid.

## PEARL OF WISDOM

The classical clinical presentation of pneumococcal pneumonia (not commonly seen these days) is of a rigor, then fever, quickly followed by pleuritic pain. Be wary because the radiographic abnormalities may lag behind the clinical presentation by several hours, and an early radiograph may be normal, causing the uninitiated to miss the diagnosis.

Malignant pleural effusions can be painful but, more commonly, they present with breathlessness. Mesothelioma is responsible for both pain and breathlessness, and the latter commonly dominates the clinical picture in the early stages when repeated fluid accumulation can be a major problem.

### 'White-out'

I use this term to describe homogeneous radio-density of one or other hemithorax. It is vitally important to ascertain whether this is as a result of massive accumulation of pleural fluid (Fig. 5.3) or, alternatively, if it is secondary to total lung collapse (Fig. 5.4). This is determined, of course, by the direction of mediastinal shift.

## HAZARD

It is vital to differentiate collapse from effusion. There have been tragic instances when the interpretation of 'white-out' has been incorrect and an intercostal drain has been inserted into a collapsed lung. This can be a fatal mistake.

### Loculation

Loculated pleural fluid tends to be a feature of empyema. It also develops if aspiration or drainage has been partially successful or if fluid reaccumulates after such intervention and pleural adhesions have formed. The inexorable progression

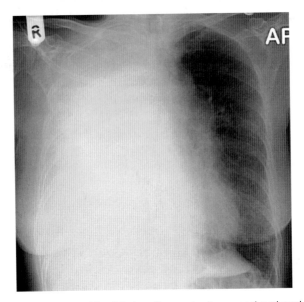

**Figure 5.3** 'White-out' of the right hemithorax due to a massive pleural effusion. A primary lung adenocarcinoma was responsible and the mediastinum is forced to the left. The right main bronchus is arrowed.

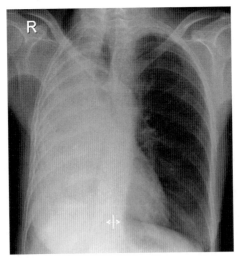

**Figure 5.4** Complete collapse of the right lung in a lady who had carcinoma of the bronchus. The mediastinal shift is obvious, and the trachea is considerably deviated to the abnormal side.

of malignant mesothelioma commonly sees pleural fluid progressively replaced by solid tumour and the pleural surface can then develop a characteristically 'lumpy' appearance.

## CLINICAL CONSIDERATIONS

Empyemata require effective drainage and seeking the early opinion of a thoracic surgeon is usually prudent.

## Haemothorax and chylothorax

It is worth considering the causes of intrapleural accumulation of both blood and chyle.

- **Haemothorax** complicates trauma and this includes iatrogenic trauma. Significantly 'bloody' effusions also occur with malignant conditions and sometimes in association with pulmonary emboli.
- **Chylothorax** results from leakage of chyle from the thoracic duct. This can be congenital, probably because the thoracic duct is absent or atretic. It can occur following intrathoracic surgery or as a result of non-surgical trauma. The latter are usually penetrating injuries but chylothorax has been reported after non-penetrating injury, e.g. hyperextension of the spine or even after violent coughing or vomiting. Non-traumatic chylothorax is usually a complication of malignant disease involving the mediastinum.

## PEARL OF WISDOM

Chylothorax: rare, non-traumatic causes include:

- yellow-nail syndrome
- lymphangioleiomyomatosis
- tuberculosis
- filariasis
- thrombosis of the jugular and subclavian veins.

## Pleural tumours

Benign pleural fibroma is a rare condition. Figure 5.5 is the chest radiograph of a 28-year-old lady who had lymphangioleiomyomatosis. The pleural lesion on the left proved to be a benign fibroma.

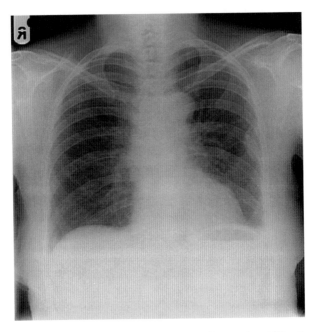

**Figure 5.5** This 28-year-old lady had a pleural fibroma in addition to lymphangioleiomyomatosis.

## Mesothelioma

A thorough industrial history is important when investigating pleural disease. Remember that the average latent period between first exposure to asbestos and death from mesothelioma is between 20 and 40 years, the variation probably being explained by the particular industry and the fibre types involved. Indeed, in a UK study reported in 1967, a latent period of less than 20 years was uncommon. The risk of developing mesothelioma is not proportional to the length or heaviness of the reported asbestos exposure, and these facts emphasize the importance of taking a careful industrial history.

For obvious reasons, mesothelioma is more common in men. It usually presents with dull chest pain (although pain can be severe and pleuritic) and breathlessness. The latter relates to the presence of pleural fluid. In the later stages of the disease, severe pain may result from invasion of thoracic nerve roots. The tumour also has a proclivity for growing out through the chest wall along the tracks of any instrumentation – a complication that is especially unpleasant. The chest radiograph usually shows a pleural effusion at first, but pleural thickening may be visible above the fluid before or after aspiration. As the tumour progresses the pleura develops a characteristically lobulated outline (Fig. 5.6). Advanced disease brings marked contraction of the affected hemithorax. The radiograph commonly also bears evidence of non-malignant pulmonary or pleural complications of asbestos exposure, as shown in Fig. 5.6.

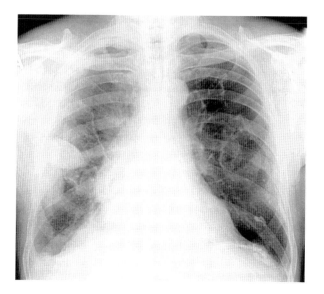

**Figure 5.6** The lobulated pleural appearance of right-sided malignant mesothelioma. There are typical calcified asbestos plaques as well, including some on the hemidiaphragms.

## Secondary tumours

Malignant conditions can invade the pleura secondarily.
Figure 5.7 appears to be an intrapulmonary lesion on the
postero-anterior radiograph. In fact it is an expanding malignant
lesion, which has destroyed much of the left second rib and has
invaded the pleura. This was a deposit of malignant myeloma.

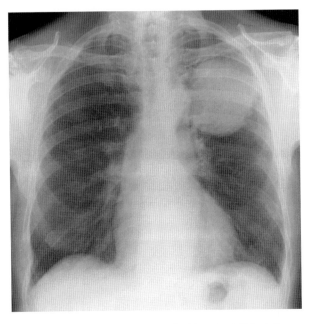

**Figure 5.7** Myeloma in a 77-year-old male. Note the left 2nd rib
destruction.

The multiple lesions apparent on Fig. 5.8 also lie within pleura,
although this is again difficult to ascertain on chest radiograph.
This is a very rare example of transcoelomic spread from a
malignant thymoma, a pattern of local spread that thymomas
can manifest. The primary tumour can be seen as an anterior
mediastinal mass, which is also spreading upwards to the
superior mediastinum. (Both the primary and secondary
tumours in this lady responded well for a time to chemotherapy.)

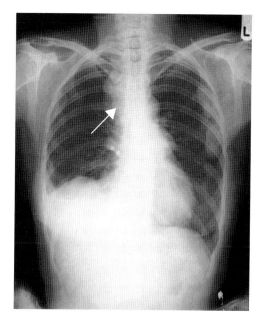

**Figure 5.8** Secondary deposits within the pleura from a malignant thymoma. Note the anterior/superior mediastinal mass, arrowed.

# PLEURAL CALCIFICATION

There are three main causes of pleural calcification:

- **calcified asbestos plaques:** the characteristic 'holly-leaf' pattern is illustrated in Figs 1.19 and 1.20 (pages 16 and 17, respectively) and the other pathognomonic feature, calcification on the hemidiaphragms, is also well illustrated. Given these appearances there should be little problem in making the diagnosis from the chest radiograph.
- tuberculosis: Fig. 5.9 is a fairly typical appearance of an old calcified tuberculous empyema. The pattern of calcification is quite different compared with asbestos plaques. What is totally unmistakeable on chest radiography is the hallmark 'en cuirasse' calcification demonstrated by

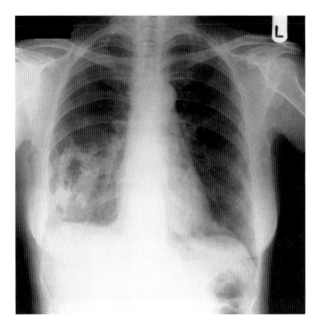

**Figure 5.9** Typical pattern of pleural calcification created by an old, healed tuberculous empyema. Calcified nodules of healed intrapulmonary tuberculosis are seen in both upper zones.

a previous artificial pneumothorax (Fig. 5.10). The calcification is again produced by healing within a tuberculous empyema.

● **previous haemothorax:** the only example I have is Fig. 5.11, which is the radiograph of a man who was a boxer in his younger days. An old healed fracture can just about be made out laterally in the left tenth rib but the small patch of calcification in the adjacent pleura is clearly seen. Any sort of trauma can result in this type of pleural calcification, but when these appearances are bilateral and multiple you can be fairly sure that you are looking at the chest radiograph of an ex-boxer.

The next chapter perfectly illustrates the importance of combining clinical and radiographic observations when managing acutely ill patients. A salutary tale is also included.

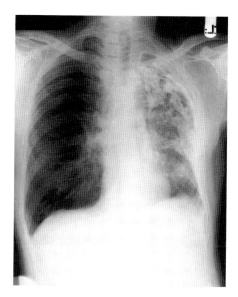

**Figure 5.10** Another, classical tuberculous empyema. This one followed artificial pneumothorax therapy.

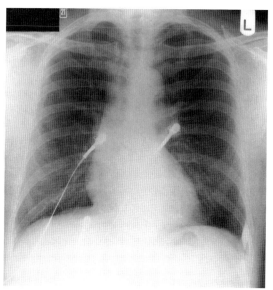

**Figure 5.11** Localized pleural calcification (left base) as a result of trauma many years previously.

# 6

# THE HYPOXAEMIC PATIENT WITH A NORMAL CHEST RADIOGRAPH

Breathlessness is one of the commonest presenting complaints of emergency medical patients. Moreover, the breathless patient who has a normal chest radiograph constitutes a common clinical scenario for those of us in acute medicine. I have taught on this topic many times largely to illustrate the common mistake of accepting the easy diagnoses of 'chest infection' or 'hyperventilation' in this scenario. These patients deserve far more thought than this because a number of important pathologies cause breathlessness without announcing themselves on a chest radiograph, and one diagnosis in particular, if missed, can result in sudden death.

In this chapter we are going to consider three groups of conditions, pulmonary vascular disease (particularly of thromboembolic aetiology), airway diseases and a heterogeneous mix of pathologies causing alveolitis, which may not be detectable on a plain radiograph in their early stages of development.

First, though, we have to engage in some basic pulmonary physiology and, despite the title of this book, I make no apology for this! Let's follow the diagnostic steps in managing the breathless patient with a normal radiograph.

## STEP ONE

Is your patient hypoxaemic as well as breathless? In most emergency departments these days, arterial oxygen saturation will be measured as a routine and a significant proportion of breathless patients will have arterial blood gases taken as well. In my experience, though, the interpretation of these tests is seldom complete. Let's take an example and consider a 23-year-old, breathless woman whose arterial oxygen saturation ($S_aO_2$) breathing air is 96 per cent.

Reassured?

You shouldn't be because, given the shape of the oxygen dissociation curve, this $S_aO_2$ can be achieved with an arterial oxygen tension ($P_aO_2$) certainly as low as 10 kPa, a level that is far from normal in a 23-year-old person. Fortunately, you are wise to this fact and you check blood gases as well. These reveal a $P_aO_2$ of 12.5 kPa, an arterial carbon dioxide tension ($P_aCO_2$) of 3 kPa and a pH 7.49.

Are you now reassured having found an oxygen tension in the normal range and a low $P_aCO_2$? Surely the patient is hyperventilating?

Wrong!

My point is that consideration of arterial oxygen tension on its own is inadequate. It must be examined in relation to what is happening in the alveolar space. In the example quoted, the $P_aCO_2$ is low. We all know that carbon dioxide transport from pulmonary capillary to lung alveolus is highly efficient and it follows that alveolar carbon dioxide tension ($P_ACO_2$) is effectively the same as the arterial partial pressure of carbon dioxide – in this case 3 kPa. The total alveolar pressure, however, must equal the atmospheric pressure, and if the carbon dioxide component falls, the contribution from another gas must rise in compensation. The nitrogen component is constant, so, in normal situations this only leaves oxygen to make up for the deficit. With this knowledge we can infer from the example quoted that alveolar oxygen tension ($P_AO_2$) should be higher than 12 kPa but we need to be more precise and measure it – the calculation is really easy and is based on the modified alveolar gas equation:

$$P_AO_2 = P_IO_2 - P_ACO_2/R$$

where $R$ is the respiratory quotient – 0.8 under most conditions – and $P_IO_2$ (the partial pressure of inspired oxygen when breathing air) is 21 per cent of atmospheric pressure so, allowing for saturated water vapour pressure, this is 21 per cent of 94.5 kPa, that is 19.845 kPa (20 for simplicity).

With the quoted example, therefore:

$$P_AO_2 = 20 - 3/0.8$$

$$P_AO_2 = 16.25 \text{ kPa}$$

This translates into an alveolar–arterial (A–a) oxygen gradient of 3.75 kPa. I would question a gradient of more than 2 kPa in a 23-year-old and would certainly be unhappy with a reading of more than 3 kPa. In other words, with a very simple calculation, our clinical concern for this young woman is heightened and this is vitally important as we shall see.

---

## ? THINKING POINT

The above equation is 'modified' because it ignores the fact that we consume a larger volume of oxygen than we produce of carbon dioxide. Therefore, with each respiratory cycle the inspired volume of alveolar gas is slightly greater than the expired volume and this is reflected in the full alveolar gas equation. In practice, when calculating $P_AO_2$ using the modified method, the inherent error is only a fraction of a kilopascal, which can be ignored in most clinical situations.

## STEP TWO

This is a short but important step. Consider these blood gases: $P_aO_2$ 16.5 kPa, $P_aCO_2$ 2 kPa, pH 7.37.

The A–a gradient calculates out at 1 kPa, which is completely normal. Presumably then, this patient is hyperventilating. Absolutely correct, but one further piece of information is crucial in order to ascertain if this is an appropriate ventilatory response to a clinical problem, namely, metabolic acidaemia. The message is simple, though often ignored – always consider the standard base excess (SBE).

 **HAZARD**

The example I have quoted is a real one, the 19-year-old student in question was thought to be a primary hyper-ventilator, her tinnitus was misinterpreted and her SBE of −9 was overlooked initially. Fortunately, the oversight was soon recognized because she was suffering from reactive depression and had taken a hefty salicylate overdose.

## STEP THREE: PULMONARY VASCULAR DISEASE

The physiological steps just covered are essential but let's move on now to consider the assessment of the patient who has an abnormal A–a oxygen gradient but no obvious explanation for this on their chest radiograph.

Figure 6.1 is the chest radiograph of a 60-year-old lady who was referred to us one evening last year with a history of sudden onset of breathlessness. She had an A–a gradient of 8 kPa, was breathless at rest and very frightened. There were no abnormal respiratory findings on examination and her radiograph, as you can see, was quite unremarkable. We anticoagulated her and organized a computerized tomography pulmonary angiogram (CTPA) – one of the images of which is reproduced in Fig. 6.2.

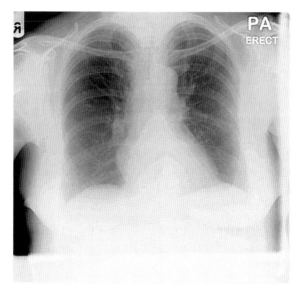

**Figure 6.1** Chest radiograph of a 60-year-old lady with sudden-onset breathlessness.

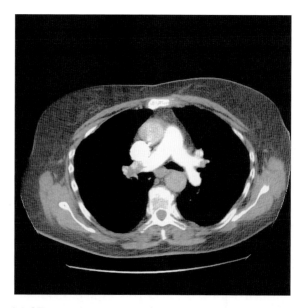

**Figure 6.2** CT scan of the patient in Fig. 6.1.

The enormous thrombus in right pulmonary artery is clearly visible. At presentation, this lady did offer some clues of pulmonary vascular pathology in that she had an elevated venous pressure and a right-sided 3rd heart sound, but never forget that major pulmonary emboli can be present in the absence of any abnormal cardiovascular or respiratory system signs. What's more, the chest radiograph and the electrocardiogram (ECG) may be normal as well.

The fundamental message is that **the default diagnosis in a patient with a normal chest radiograph and hypoxaemia is that of pulmonary embolism.**

It is essential to cover this possibility with anticoagulant therapy while you confirm or refute the diagnosis – pulmonary thromboembolic disease is potentially fatal and if one embolism has occurred there may well be another one waiting to happen.

There are a number of important and interesting clinical points to make:

 **CLINICAL CONSIDERATIONS**

Major pulmonary embolism may not be accompanied by abnormal clinical findings. However, when there are abnormalities these can manifest as follows:

● evidence of compromised cardiac output with hypotension and cold, clammy peripheries, with or without a sinus tachycardia
● signs of pulmonary hypertension with an elevated jugular venous pressure (JVP) (perhaps with a particularly prominent 'A' wave), a loud pulmonary second heart sound and a right parasternal heave indicative of right ventricular hypertrophy.

Either group of signs may dominate.

Electrocardiographic observations are important too:

- the classical (and often quoted) abnormality is that of 'S1, Q3, T3'. This isn't as common as some books would have you believe and isn't specific for pulmonary vascular disease either
- the changes are often much more subtle – right bundle branch block with or without a broad QRS complex, S–T segment or T-wave change inferiorly, or evidence of right ventricular strain with T-wave inversion in the anteroseptal leads

**However, there is a classical trap here. Don't fall into it.** The sudden insult to the right ventricle provided by the sudden increase in right ventricular afterload created by a major pulmonary embolism results in an increased demand for oxygen and, therefore, coronary blood flow by the struggling right ventricle. This may translate into electrocardiographic changes that are predominantly left-sided, particularly if the patient has existing coronary artery disease and blood flow is diverted away from an already compromised left ventricular blood supply. The clinical corollary to this is that major pulmonary embolism regularly causes cardiac chest pain and can even result in 'secondary' myocardial damage. This is recognized more commonly these days with the advent of troponin assay and the observation that this cardio-specific enzyme is regularly elevated in pulmonary embolic disease.

 **HAZARD**

It is vital to remember that a normal ECG in no way excludes the diagnosis of pulmonary embolism.

**THINKING POINT**

Smaller pulmonary emboli tend to present with pleurisy perhaps because they are able to reach the periphery of the lung and involve the pleura. Large emboli, on the other hand, are regularly painless and present with breathlessness and/or haemodynamic abnormalities. The absence of pleurisy **does not** exclude pulmonary embolism and, remember, size isn't everything – a small embolus may well not cause you harm whereas the large one, which is waiting to follow it, may prove fatal.

## The abnormal radiograph in pulmonary embolism

For completeness sake we should consider the radiographic abnormalities that can accompany pulmonary thromboembolic disease, not least because these radiographic signs may be very subtle.

- One or other (and occasionally both) hemidiaphragms may be elevated.
- There may be line shadows at the bases.

Either of these observations should cause you to question the diagnostic possibility of thromboembolic disease.

- One or other main pulmonary artery may be bulky, directly reflecting the presence of clot within it. This is usually seen on the right side but only because the right pulmonary artery is not obscured by heart shadow.
- Westermark's sign is an area of hypoperfusion somewhere in the lung fields and is very uncommon. In fact at least one of my radiological colleagues does not believe that it exists – I think Fig. 6.3 proves him wrong though!

Figure 6.4 is a detail of the CTPA of the same patient. There is an enormous amount of thrombus bilaterally. This man, happily, made an excellent recovery with thrombolysis.

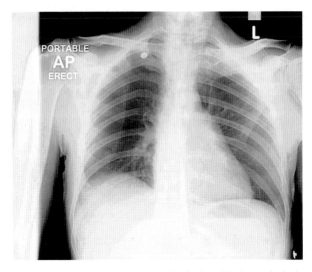

**Figure 6.3** Both pulmonary arteries are bulky but this is particularly obvious on the right where it is accompanied by a beautiful example of Westermark's sign.

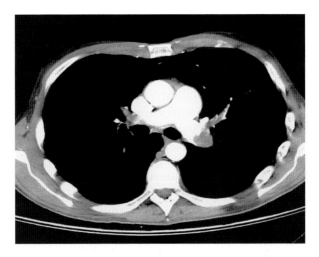

**Figure 6.4** Computerized tomography pulmonary angiogram of the same patient as in Fig. 6.3.

## Other types of pulmonary vascular disease

- **Secondary pulmonary hypertension** often occurs as a result of chronic obstructive pulmonary disease. The cardinal radiographic appearances are those of bilateral enlargement of proximal pulmonary arteries and peripheral vascular attenuation. There may be ancillary radiographic evidence of pulmonary pathology and the bullous change illustrated in Fig. 1.23 (page 19) is an example.
- **Idiopathic pulmonary hypertension** produces the same vascular appearances. Clinically, the presentation tends to be one of progressive rather than acute dyspnoea.

---

**?** **THINKING POINT**

The default diagnosis of the hypoxaemic patient with a normal chest radiograph is that of pulmonary embolism. There are other diagnostic possibilities but pulmonary embolism can be multiple and it can be fatal. Unless there is another explanation for this presentation, your patient should be anticoagulated while the diagnosis is excluded, either by CTPA or ventilation–perfusion lung scan. If the clinical features include significant cardiovascular abnormalities or severe hypoxaemia it is the author's view that CTPA is the investigation of choice, not least because thrombolysis of the blood clot may be necessary and its direct visualization will assist in making this decision.

---

## STEP FOUR: AIRWAY DISEASES

A disease process that predominantly affects airways will produce a ventilation–perfusion mismatch and therefore an abnormal A–a oxygen gradient. The pathology may well not be visible on the chest radiograph, however. There are a few salient points in relation to specific diseases.

- **Asthma:** asthmatic patients may indeed be severely hypoxaemic with nothing to show on the radiograph. However, there should be no problem in diagnosing an acute asthmatic since the clinical findings are so obvious. The challenge is to recognize just how severe the attack is, and objective measurements, especially those of gas exchange, are vital in this regard; clinical quantifiers of severity are simply not reliable.

- **Smoking-related airways obstruction:** chronic bronchitis and emphysema also disrupt the ventilation–perfusion relationship and although there may be radiographic abnormalities, bullae, abnormal vascular distribution or evidence of pulmonary hypertension, the radiographic changes may be unremarkable. Acute infective exacerbation of chronic obstructive pulmonary disease (COPD) results in further ventilation–perfusion mismatch with consequent further deterioration in hypoxaemia. The problem is that there is no way to quantify the degree of hypoxaemia that it is reasonable to see in these circumstances without having to invoke additional pathological processes as the explanation. Put very simply, there are no clinical studies that relate the degree of hypoxaemia to the amount of tobacco consumed in the stable smoker and no studies quantifying the ventilation–perfusion mismatch that may be expected in acute exacerbation in relation to the severity of the background airways disease. Add to this the fact that individuals with COPD are at risk of pulmonary thromboembolism, and the potential for mistakes is obvious. I have no magic answer to this dilemma but the fundamental approach is to be aware of the pitfalls as presented – in patients with acute exacerbations of smoking-related chronic airways disease, always look for a reason for their deterioration. Infection is the commonest explanation; an element of heart failure is common too but always consider the possibility of co-existent pulmonary embolism.

- **Acute bronchiolitis:** this condition is far commoner in children but can also occur in adults in whom the diagnosis is often unsuspected. A variety of common viruses may be responsible and the clinical findings are of a breathless patient, commonly pyrexial, with a history suggestive of respiratory tract infection and who may be severely hypoxaemic despite having a normal chest X-ray. If physical signs are present these are commonly inspiratory crackles, although high-pitched wheezes ('squawks') may be heard also. Be alert to the diagnosis, because corticosteroid therapy is often indicated.

- **Other airway diseases:** I cannot resist the temptation of showing the images of a young woman who was admitted through our department about 18 months ago (Figs 6.5 and 6.6). She was breathless and severely hypoxaemic and although her radiograph is not entirely normal (it does show a degree of hyperinflation), the clinical and physiological abnormalities were far out of proportion to

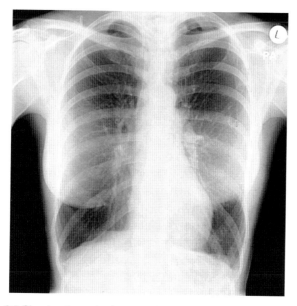

**Figure 6.5** Chest radiograph of a young lady with obliterative bronchiolitis.

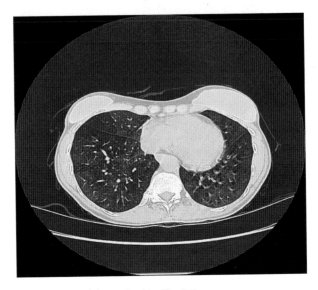

**Figure 6.6** CT scan of the patient in Fig. 6.5.

the radiographic change. The CT scan (Fig. 6.6 shows an image taken in expiration) reveals marked air-trapping in lung parenchyma. This young woman has obliterative bronchiolitis, a condition associated with rheumatoid arthritis and other collagen vascular diseases although apparently idiopathic in this case.

## STEP FIVE: ALVEOLITIDES

Finally, a wide variety of conditions, which result in alveolitis or an alveolar-filling process may cause dramatic disruption to gas exchange at a time when the chest radiograph is apparently normal. It is important to be aware of this because the most discriminative clue to the presence of these conditions is often the history and this is illustrated by the following real examples of patients who have been admitted through our acute medical unit over the past 12 months. All of these patients had normal chest radiographs.

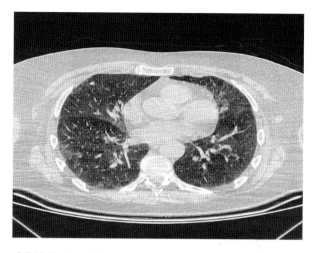

**Figure 6.7** Methotrexate lung.

Figure 6.7 is a CT image of a 68-year-old lady with rheumatoid arthritis. The CT scan was requested in view of her history of methotrexate therapy and is highly abnormal. This is 'methotrexate lung' and the pulmonary infiltration disappeared following corticosteroid treatment.

Figure 6.8 shows a 'ground-glass' appearance on CT scan in a 30-year-old farmer. Farmers' lung is uncommon in Norfolk, probably because of the relatively dry climate, but this was an example, again responding completely to steroids.

The CT abnormalities of Fig. 6.9 are more impressive but the chest radiograph was again normal. This young man also had extrinsic allergic alveolitis – in this case 'bird-fanciers' lung. (He kept a ring-necked parakeet, the latin name for which, for those of you who enjoy such information, is *Psittacula krameri*.)

In addition, *Pneumocystis carinii* pneumonia is well documented as presenting with dyspnoea and hypoxia in the presence of a normal chest radiograph and the same is reported in desquamative interstial pneumonitis.

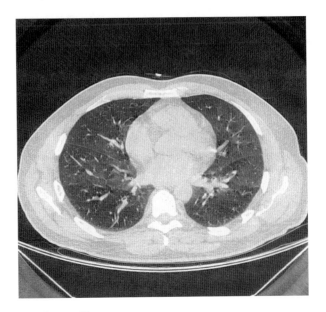

**Figure 6.8** Farmers' lung.

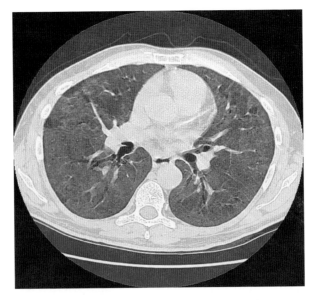

**Figure 6.9** Bird (specifically *Psittacula krameri*!) fanciers' lung.

## ? THINKING POINT

The fundamental learning point is to be aware of these possibilities and to question their existence through comprehensive history-taking and clinical examination. Hypoxaemia with a normal chest radiograph is a clinical scenario hiding many pathological possibilities other than simply 'chest infection'.

# 7

# PRACTICE EXAMPLES AND 'FASCINOMAS'

This final chapter comprises a series of interesting chest radiographs on which to practise the diagnostic skills I have described, and it concludes with some fascinating cases that I have encountered over the years. The latter films are instructive in their own right and they are not just an excuse for me to indulge in middle-aged nostalgia – although there may be a smattering of this!

## PRACTICE EXAMPLES

Examine the radiographs that follow (each of them is accompanied by short clinical notes), follow the investigative approach described in earlier chapters and take time to record **all** of the abnormalities. Then make an attempt at a diagnosis and check your observations and diagnosis with the answers that follow.

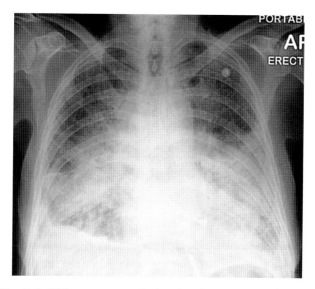

- **Fig. 7.1:** This man was admitted to hospital with severe breathlessness.

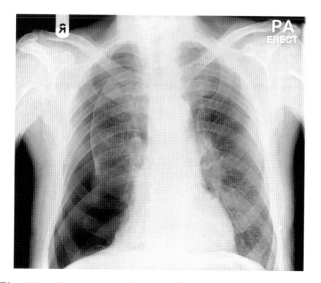

- **Fig. 7.2:** An easy one this but there is a lot of information to collect – don't overlook any of it.

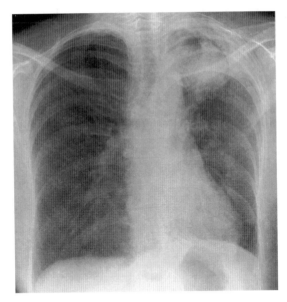

● Fig. 7.3: Haemoptysis was the presenting complaint here.

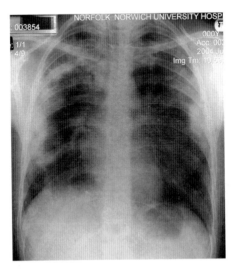

● Fig. 7.4: This young man had been unwell for two weeks before this radiograph was taken – his symptoms were fever, cough and severe general malaise. Note the distribution of the abnormal pulmonary shadowing.

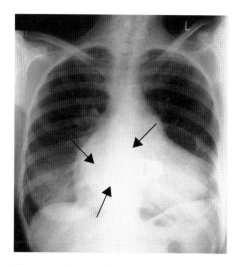

- Fig. 7.5: There are lots of abnormalities on this radiograph and they come together to tell quite a story about this woman who suffered rheumatic fever in childhood.

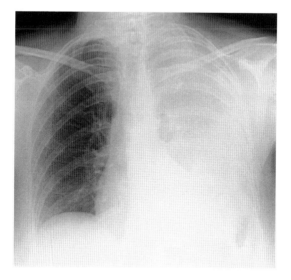

- Fig. 7.6: Weight loss and fever were the presenting complaints and this lady was severely cachectic when she finally came to hospital. How will you manage the problem?

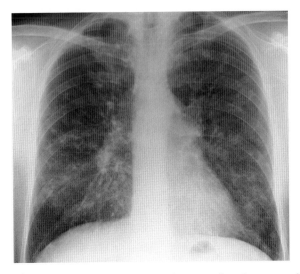

● **Fig. 7.7:** This late teenager has been under the care of the chest clinic since early childhood.

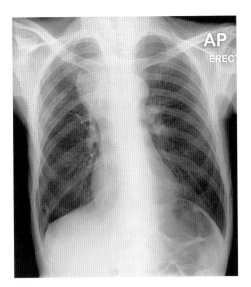

● **Fig. 7.8:** The radiographic abnormalities were a fortuitous finding in this young man who presented with weight loss and chest pain when imbibing alcohol.

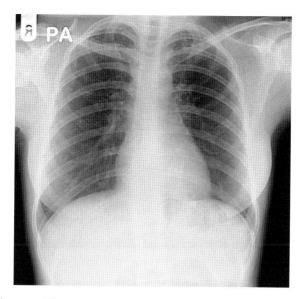

● Fig. 7.9: The presenting complaints were night sweats and weight loss in this lady from the Phillipines.

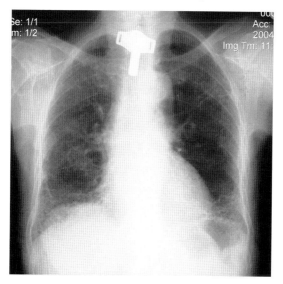

● Fig. 7.10: Full marks if you can put all of the abnormalities together to make a diagnosis here.

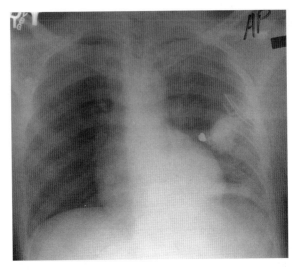

- Fig. 7.11: Have a shot at this diagnosis.

## ANSWERS

- Fig. 7.1: Pulmonary infiltration is peri-hilar in distribution and has coalesced to produce an alveolar-filling pattern. It is impossible to comment on heart size but there is pleural fluid, certainly on the right. The intrapulmonary shadowing is too dense to see septal lines but the most likely diagnosis is left ventricular failure. Other possibilities exist, however, and these include alveolar haemorrhage, adult respiratory distress syndrome, *Pneumocystis* pneumonia and pulmonary alveolar proteinosis.

- Fig. 7.2: No prizes for diagnosing the right-sided pneumothorax, but note the complete collapse of the right lower lobe, the thickened visceral pleura (the pneumothorax had probably occurred a week earlier from the history) and the bilaterally prominent proximal pulmonary vessels. There is no significant mediastinal shift. This man had been a lifelong smoker, he had associated chronic airways obstruction and pulmonary hypertension and a bulla in the right lower lobe had leaked. He required surgical pleurodesis when the pneumothorax failed to re-inflate with an intercostal drain.

- **Fig. 7.3:** This is a classic radiograph. There is fibrosis and loss of volume in the left upper lobe and the lesion at the left apex can be seen to be a cavity with a mass contained within it. The halo sign is evident and the pleural thickening at the apex makes it 'full-house' for the diagnosis of aspergilloma. Speckled intrapulmonary shadowing is evident in the right mid-zone and this strongly suggests tuberculosis as the original cause of the fibrosis and cavitation. Haemoptysis can be dramatic in this condition, as it was in this case.

- **Fig. 7.4:** The clue to the diagnosis is the peripheral distribution of the consolidation. This is an example of eosinophilic pneumonia. The typical radiographic appearances facilitated a prompt diagnosis, and complete radiographic resolution quickly accrued with corticosteroid therapy.

- **Fig. 7.5:** A ring of calcium can be seen behind the heart (arrows). The left atrial wall has become calcified in response to long-standing elevation in left atrial pressure as a result of mitral stenosis. The rib changes compatible with a left lateral thoracotomy can be seen and this lady underwent a closed mitral valvotomy before her median sternotomy (note the wire sternal sutures) and mitral valve replacement with a Starr–Edwards prosthesis several years later.

- **Fig. 7.6:** There is a 'white-out' of the left lung with some mediastinal shift to the opposite side – evidence of a large pleural effusion. A diagnostic pleural tap produced pus, and an intercostal drain was inserted into this massive empyema. Formal surgical drainage was subsequently required.

- **Fig. 7.7:** The salient radiographic features are multiple 'blotchy' shadows, linear shadows, toothpaste shadows and occasional tramlines, all in association with some cystic spaces. This combination of abnormalities is highly suggestive of bronchiectasis and this young person has cystic fibrosis.

- Fig. 7.8: The differential diagnosis of superior mediastinal masses has been discussed in Chapter 2. Mediastinoscopy and biopsy in this case resulted in a diagnosis of Hodgkin's disease.
- Fig. 7.9: There are abnormal nodules particularly in the upper zones. In a patient from the Far East this is tuberculosis until proved otherwise and this suspicion was confirmed on sputum microscopy.
- Fig. 7.10: The reticulo-nodular infiltrate is fairly generalized although still perhaps with a discernible predominance in the lower zones and peripherally elsewhere. There is localized honeycombing and fibrosing alveolitis is the likely diagnosis. You will have noted subluxation of the right shoulder joint, and the problem here was rheumatoid-associated interstitial fibrosis. The tracheostomy was necessitated by severe upper airway obstruction due to a combination of tracheomalacia and rheumatoid involvement of the crico-arytenoid joints.
- Fig. 7.11: Apologies for the pun in the clue, this is a gunshot wound. The bullet is in the lung with an area of adjacent pulmonary haemorrhage.

## FASCINOMAS

I thought it would be fun to conclude with some unusual cases I have encountered over the years. Hopefully, these will whet your appetite for the fascinating radiographic diagnoses that are waiting for you around the corner. Keep your eyes open, observe and record systematically and you will find them.

### Figure 7.12

Another example of this fabulous X-ray may not be waiting around the corner, representing as it does a long-extinct surgical technique for the treatment of tuberculosis. The speckled calcification, particularly in the right upper zone, gives away the primary diagnosis. The multiple rounded opacities at the left apex appear to reside within the pleural space and indeed they do. This is an example of 'plombage'. Spheres of an early

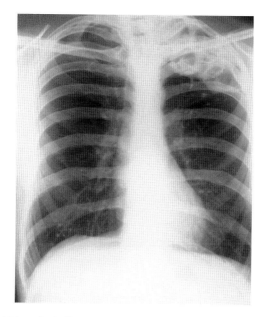

**Figure 7.12** Leucite balls.

plastic called leucite were placed in the pleural cavity in an attempt to create permanent collapse of lung infected with *Mycobacterium tuberculosis* – an organism that does not tolerate poor ventilation. Note the spelling of 'leucite', I remember a registrar in Cardiff (who shall remain nameless) who, mistakenly, described them as 'lewisite' balls – the treatment, though fairly harsh, was not as explosive as that!

## Figure 7.13(a) and (b)

These are the postero-anterior (p–a) and lateral views, respectively of a child who was the son of a sheep farmer in West Wales.

That should give the diagnosis away!

Note the halo sign in the enormous cavity. This was a pulmonary hydatid cyst.

## Figure 7.14(a) and (b)

A 32-year-old Indonesian sailor docked in Cardiff some years ago and promptly attended the chest clinic there. With some

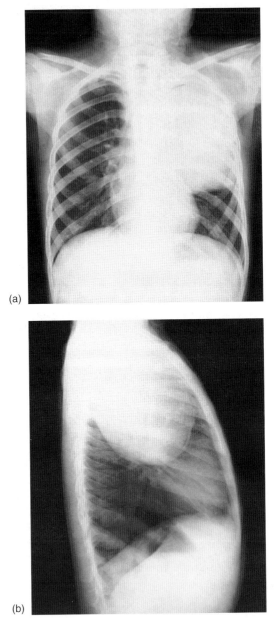

(a)

(b)

**Figure 7.13** (a) Hydatid cyst, postero-anterior view. (b) Hydatid cyst, lateral view.

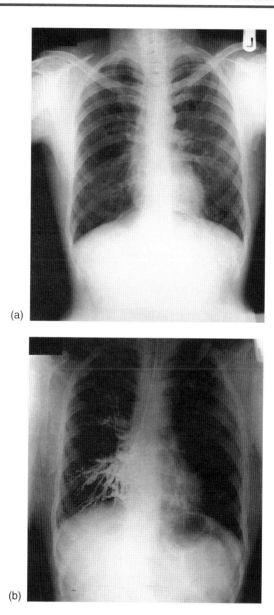

(a)

(b)

**Figure 7.14** (a) and (b) Paragonimiasis.

difficulty (because his English was poor) we finally elicited a history of weight loss and haemoptysis. Cystic lesions can be seen on his radiograph but these aren't terribly striking. Nevertheless, Brian Davies (my boss at the time) made the stunning diagnosis of paragonimiasis. None of us believed him but he was absolutely right! The burrows of the lung fluke can be seen on the bronchogram.

> **?  THINKING POINT**
>
> *Paragonimus* has a complicated life cycle, which involves a freshwater snail, shell-fish and human hosts at different stages. Humans usually become infected by ingesting raw shell-fish and there is a favoured dish in Indonesia, apparently, which is called 'drunken crab'.
>
> This dish appeared to have been the source of the infection in this case. 'Drunken crab' is raw crab doused in alcohol, not as one of the registrars at the time (a different one) believed it to be and I quote, 'Is that a crab that walks in a straight line, Brian?'.

## Figure 7.15

This is an X-ray of a Chinese child. The right paratracheal lymphadenopathy is clearly seen and was a manifestation of primary pulmonary tuberculosis. Note the mediastinal shift to the opposite side and this is accompanied by obstructive emphysema of the right lung. Presumably this structural change was made possible by the immature stage of development of this child's airways.

## Figure 7.16

This man had worked as a coal miner in Germany under appalling conditions for some years culminating in 1950 when he emigrated to this country. He then worked at the coal-face in the Nottinghamshire coal-field and had a series of

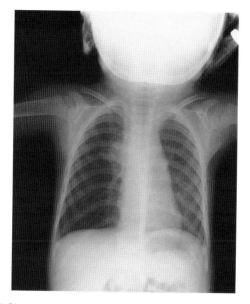

**Figure 7.15** Obstructive emphysema.

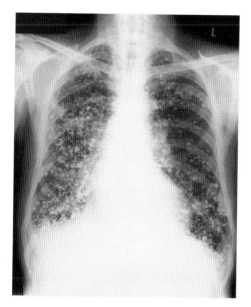

**Figure 7.16** Amyloidosis.

radiographs performed from the early 1960s until this film – taken in 1978. His functional disability was relatively slight despite the fact that the radiographs showed progressive calcification of initially faint nodulation over the years. The diagnosis had always been a puzzle, the slow progression and the nature of the calcification not really fitting with any clear diagnosis. His rheumatoid factor was negative and there was no support for an unusual case of Caplan's syndrome, there was no fibrosis and anyway the shadows aren't correct for silicosis – so this case was altogether a mystery and was explained away as an unusual type of pneumoconiosis, presumably related to the appalling conditions he had encountered in Germany before and during the second world war.

In 1978 he was admitted with a myocardial infarction, which unhappily proved fatal and post-mortem examination revealed extensive intrapulmonary amyloidosis. It transpired therefore that his intriguing radiographs had nothing whatsoever to do with his dust exposure.

## Figure 7.17(a) and (b)

Last but quite definitely not least, this lady was referred to me for biopsy of the 'solitary' pulmonary nodule at the left base behind the heart. Fortunately, we made two observations before wielding the biopsy needle. First, the lesion was not solitary and, secondly, she had telangiectasia on her lips.

A pulmonary angiogram was performed instead of a lung biopsy and these beautifully shown arterio-venous malformations are well recognized associations of Osler–Rendu–Weber syndrome. A biopsy would not have been a good idea.

There have been so many fascinating cases over the years that I could go on and on but I fear that the bill for illustrations would not please my publishers!

We must call a halt, therefore, and this is an appropriate case with which to conclude – emphasizing, as it does, the necessity for lateral thought and the importance of combining clinical and radiographic information when managing patients.

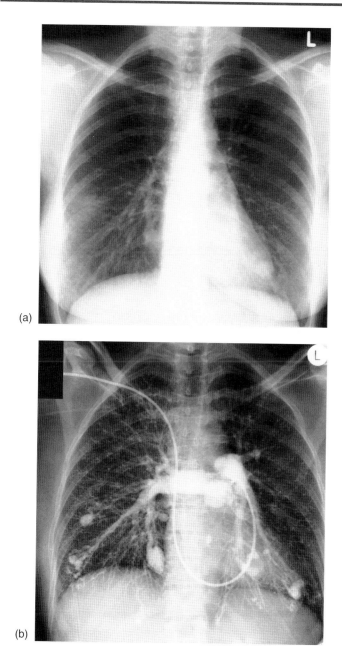

(a)

(b)

**Figure 7.17** (a) and (b) Osler–Rendu–Weber syndrome.

# FURTHER READING

The following are standard texts that I use regularly and recommend highly:

## RADIOLOGY TEXTBOOKS

Armstrong P., Wilson A. G., Dee P. and Hansell D.E. 2000:
*Imaging of diseases of the chest*, 3rd edn. London, Edinburgh, Philadelphia, St Louis, Sydney, Toronto: Mosby.
A mine of information – superb.

Simon G. 1978: *Principles of chest X-ray diagnosis*,
4th edn. London, Boston: Butterworths.
The 4th edition of this classic was published posthumously in 1978, but it should still be possible to find a second-hand copy. I think Simon's work is an absolute must for those who wish to master descriptive radiographic observation and diagnosis.

Fraser R. S., Pare P. D., Muller N. L. and Colman N. 1999:
*Diagnosis of diseases of the chest* ['Fraser and Pare'], 4th edn.
London, Edinburgh, Philadelphia, St Louis, Sydney, Toronto: Elsevier Saunders.
I bought my first copy of Fraser and Pare in Blackwells in Oxford in 1981 when I could not afford it and I have never regretted my profligacy. This is a truly fantastic book, an

incredible source of original references and is first choice to accompany me to my desert island.

# RESPIRATORY MEDICINE TEXTBOOKS

Seaton A., Douglas Seaton D. and Leitch A. G. (eds). 2000: *Crofton and Douglas's respiratory diseases,* 5th edn. Oxford: Blackwell.
A personal favourite, my original copy dates back to 1978 and has been used so much that it is virtually falling apart.

Gibson G. J., Geddes D. M, Costobel U., Sterk P. J. and Corrin B. (eds). 2003: *Respiratory medicine,* 3rd edn. London, Edinburgh, Philadelphia, St Louis, Sydney, Toronto: Saunders.
This is another brilliantly comprehensive general respiratory medicine textbook and is strongly recommended.

Murray J. F. and Nadel J. A. with Mason R. J. and Boushey H. A. 2000: *Textbook of respiratory medicine,* 3rd edn. Boston: Saunders.

Alfred P. and Fishman A. P. 1988: *Pulmonary diseases and disorders,* 2nd edn. London/New York: McGraw Hill.
The latest edition that I can find was published in 1988 (and it has been on my shelf since then!). This is another personal favourite.

# INDEX